Dynamic X-ray Imaging Systems Used in Medicine

Quality control in performance characteristics

IPEM–IOP Series in Physics and Engineering in Medicine and Biology

About the Series

The Series in Physics and Engineering in Medicine and Biology will allow IPEM to enhance its mission to 'advance physics and engineering applied to medicine and biology for the public good'.

Focusing on key areas including, but not limited to:

- clinical engineering
- diagnostic radiology
- informatics and computing
- magnetic resonance imaging
- nuclear medicine
- physiological measurement
- radiation protection
- radiotherapy
- rehabilitation engineering
- ultrasound and non-ionising radiation.

A number of IPEM–IOP titles are published as part of the EUTEMPE Network Series for Medical Physics Experts.

Dynamic X-ray Imaging Systems Used in Medicine

Quality control in performance characteristics

Edited by
Greg Stevens
University Hospital Plymouth, Plymouth, UK

IOP Publishing, Bristol, UK

ISBN 978-0-7503-3819-6 (ebook)
ISBN 978-0-7503-3817-2 (print)
ISBN 978-0-7503-3820-2 (myPrint)
ISBN 978-0-7503-3818-9 (mobi)

DOI 10.1088/978-0-7503-3819-6

Version: 20211001

IOP ebooks

British Library Cataloguing-in-Publication Data: A catalogue record for this book is available from the British Library.

Published by IOP Publishing, wholly owned by The Institute of Physics, London

IOP Publishing, Temple Circus, Temple Way, Bristol, BS1 6HG, UK

US Office: IOP Publishing, Inc., 190 North Independence Mall West, Suite 601, Philadelphia, PA 19106, USA

Contents

IPEM Report Number 32, Part VIII

A Report produced by the Institute of Physics and Engineering in Medicine

Working party members

Amber Gislason-Lee

Ben Johnson

Greg Stevens

Ian Honey

Nicholas Marshall

Peter Hiles

Chapter 1

Introduction

1.1 Scope of this report

The aim of this report is to discuss the methods and techniques that may be used to commission and perform routine quality control (QC) measurements of dynamic x-ray imaging systems. In recent years the range of interventional, and clinical procedures that are reliant on these imaging systems has grown. This has brought about an increasingly broad range of x-ray imaging equipment which can capture motion. Therefore in the context of this report the term 'dynamic x-ray imaging systems' refers to this subset of (fixed and mobile) imaging systems, whereas fluoroscopy refers to a specific mode.

Since dynamic imaging equipment is used for a wide range of clinical applications, the report includes a general description of the characteristics and operational aspects to assist the medical physicist with clinical set-up and performance evaluation strategies. In particular, the automatic dose rate control (ADRC) plays a significant role in determining the balance between patient dose and image quality; in consequence, the function and evaluation of ADRC devices is covered in detail.

QC is performed for a number of reasons: to fulfil regulatory requirements, for acceptance of testing purposes, to provide baseline data that can be used to track system performance over time, and to provide benchmark data for assessing system set-up for the tasks to be performed by the system, as well as any associated optimisation that may be required. Taken together, these steps should help to ensure that the system is set up at least adequately or even optimally for the intended task, and that there has been no change in performance that will adversely affect clinical decisions. All of this is done within the limitations of the available testing methods and test objects.

1.2 Preface

Report 32 has an illustrious history; originally published by the Hospital Physicists Association as a series of six reports in booklet form. These were revised over the

doi:10.1088/978-0-7503-3819-6ch1

years to account for new developments in equipment and practice, and proved to be a standard reference for fluoroscopy testing. However, the clinical utility of dynamic x-ray imaging systems has evolved tremendously since the introduction of the flat panel system in the year 2000.

For example, endovascular procedures are becoming more common and patient conditions that were once treated with open surgery are now treated interventionally and sent home the same day. Hybrid operating theatres where surgeons and interventional radiologists both use dynamic x-ray equipment are increasing in number across the UK. These procedures are made possible by imaging techniques such as roadmapping, digital subtraction angiography (DSA), and cone beam computed tomography (CBCT). New single-screen television (TV) monitors show considerable improvements in configuration over the older multiple monitor setup, as this single large monitor may be split into user configurable areas, to display a range of information such as previous imaging (from PACs), ultrasound traces, EEG/ECG traces, heart information etc.

With the increase of computing power over the last few decades there has been increased automation of, not only the selection of radiographic factors but also image processing options. Manufacturers are not willing to share details on how these automated functions work; this makes it increasingly difficult for physicists to understand, control, and test these imaging options.

Manufacturers can now perform dynamic image processing in real time. In some of the more complex systems, different algorithms can be separately applied to different parts of a given image frame to enhance image quality locally. While this has proved of benefit clinically, the older, static test objects featured in report 32 may have lost some relevance, and therefore may not necessarily represent the image quality that the clinician may see during a patient procedure. This in turn has led to disagreement between clinicians, physicists, and manufacturers over exactly what a QC image quality test provides, what is acceptable, and what is not.

This has been demonstrated by findings from the Evidence Based Quality Assurance (QA) Project [1], started by the IPEM Diagnostic Radiology Special Interest Group (DRSIG). Some information about the efficacy of current QC testing has been provided despite inconsistent practice across the UK and, where possible, data from the Evidence Based QA (EBQA) project has been integrated into this report.

The technology behind these systems never stands still, the systems are always evolving, and there are concerns that this report will become obsolete sooner than would be hoped. We have therefore made a number of compromises and worked together with authors of the Medical and Dental Guidance Notes (MDGN) and the IPEM EBQA publications to assure consistency.

There are likely to be advances in ADRC systems which will be driven to a greater extent by the (clinical) image content and make use of non-linear and non-stationary (i.e. local) image processing. However, we expect that the underlying performance of the x-ray tube and detector will remain vital aspects of the final, 'delivered' image quality. With the implementation of the NEMA user QC mode [2], the quantitative/physical evaluation of the x-ray tube and x-ray detector should become easier and essential fixed and firm points in the QC of the total system.

In the UK, image quality evaluation of fluoroscopy for QC purposes has generally used contrast-detail techniques and focused on the x-ray detector [3]. We expect these measures to correlate closely with physical image quality parameters of the x-ray detector (the pre-sampling modulation transfer function (MTF), noise power spectrum (NPS), the detective quantum efficiency (DQE) and the (applied/intrinsic) lag). These data can be used to track the performance of the system or components (x-ray tube, x-ray detector) over the lifetime of the system.

The difficulties arise in trying to assess the final output image quality for the myriad of fluoroscopy and acquisition modes that are programmed on these imaging systems. The challenge for QC physicists lies in making an accurate/useful measurement of the 'image quality' of the clinical images, for the chosen imaging application, where the result may depend on the test object used. It is clear that imaging performance comparisons between imaging systems (even of the same vendor) must be made with care.

The authors hope this publication provides as a minimum the knowledge required to allow physicists and technologists who are experienced in QC of x-ray equipment to undertake tests on dynamic imaging equipment, with an understanding of the methods applied, the associated limitations and compromises, and the value of the data and results they have acquired.

In line with previous parts of the IPEM report 32 series, a single report format is employed, with terminology updated to reflect the current state of the technology. A glossary is provided in the final pages. While this report is intended to give the practicing physicist the tools to adequately test a new x-ray system, it is also intended to allow testing of legacy equipment.

1.3 Rationale for the approach used

Modern imaging equipment contains an array of user selectable and automatic options that allow systems to be configured to cover a range of possible clinical applications; these options are then tailored to a specific clinical task. It should be understood that the impact on patient dose and image quality of selecting different imaging protocols can be substantial.

Furthermore, testing the system under carefully controlled conditions may not reflect the way in which the equipment performs in clinical use. The approach taken in this report is therefore to divide test methods into those used to evaluate the image detector (under controlled conditions) and those for assessing the overall system (under task-specific settings). In the latter case, it is not generally possible to test all possible permutations of equipment settings, but rather attention should be focused on a smaller number of clinical protocols used frequently on the system of interest.

1.4 What makes dynamic x-ray systems different?

It is imperative that the reader understands what makes dynamic x-ray systems different, and there are several important factors. This section therefore introduces this x-ray system type to readers who are less familiar with it.

Modern dynamic imaging systems are used to visualise the motion of human anatomy, internal fluids, and clinical devices inside a patient by acquiring sequences of image frames. These systems are used in a wide range of clinical applications and it is therefore of the utmost importance to understand the clinical purpose and operation of the dynamic imaging system before commencing testing. Systems that are nominally the same may be set up in very different ways for different clinical procedures and therefore some knowledge of the intended use is required before acceptance or routine QC tests are performed.

There are a large number of competing system characteristics that must be balanced in order to ensure a system has the required temporal resolution (to accurately visualise motion), spatial resolution (to visualise small devices), minimised image noise, optimised patient dose, and that intrinsic x-ray system power or heating limits are not exceeded.

In order to meet these expectations manufacturers employ a feedback loop, which automatically adjusts a number of system parameters such that the resulting 'image quality' is sufficient for the operator to perform the clinical task in question. This is termed the automatic dose rate control (ADRC) in this report; see section 2.2 for a detailed description. This is different from the automatic exposure control used in radiography, where built-in radiation detectors measure the image detector dose and cut off radiation output when a predetermined dose has been acquired.

Although different manufacturers have differing ADRC design mechanisms, they all seek to meet the same requirements. Patient thickness and body habitus, which are projection-angle dependent, and the level of image quality set by the imaging mode dictate how the ADRC sets the peak tube voltage, peak tube current (often referred to as 'mA'), and x-ray frame (i.e. pulse) duration; in some cases spectral x-ray beam filtration and focal spot size can also be altered dynamically.

Broadly, there are two main types of imaging mode supported by dynamic imaging systems. 'Fluoroscopy' is the dynamic mode in which a sequence of images are generated and displayed in real time for 'live' visualisation during a clinical procedure, and is predominantly used to visualise interventional devices, contrast medium, or anatomy in real time for diagnostic uses. If desired, the fluoroscopy run can often be stored for later review (usually called 'fluorograb' or 'fluorostore' using manufacturer terminology).

The second mode is 'acquisition' in which the images are stored during the sequence and can be reviewed during or after the procedure for diagnosis or treatment assessment. Acquisition modes can be set up to produce single images (referred to as 'spot imaging' in the past), cineradiography ('cine') for cardiac imaging, and image sequences with or without temporal subtraction of a mask image, i.e. DSA.

The original name 'cine' was given because the earlier generation of image intensifier television (IITV) based systems used photographic film for image storage. However, all solid state flat panel (FP) detector based x-ray systems utilise the same detector for image capture in both fluoroscopy and acquisition modes. For modern dynamic imaging systems, including modern II systems, the term 'acquisition' is more appropriate and is therefore used in place of 'cine' or 'fluorography' throughout this report.

DSA is used in neurological and vascular imaging to acquire images with unwanted background anatomy subtracted, in order to reveal finely detailed vascular structures. In 'roadmapping' modes a DSA image is superimposed on a live fluoroscopy run. As a generalisation, the detector air KERMA (DAK) per frame is lowest for fluoroscopy modes, higher for acquisition modes, and highest for DSA applications, to meet the image quality levels demanded in these applications. However, some vascular-specific systems whose most commonly used mode is DSA or roadmapping employ lower dose, fluoroscopy based, or 'blended' DSA.

When using dynamic imaging systems the operator selects the most appropriate imaging mode for the clinical task, adjusts the field of view, magnification, collimation, patient table height, and other settings such as x-ray source to image detector distance (SID). There are a variety of methods used for initiating an exposure. For interventional and large cardiac systems the operator generally has two foot pedals for hands-free operation—one pedal for each of two operating modes. For diagnostic cases a single pedal or hand switch for fluoroscopy is provided together with a means to store the currently shown image of a fluoroscopy run. It is important to realise that on some systems the operation of both hand switches and pedals can be programmed.

When fluoroscopy exposure is initiated the first few frames are used by the ADRC system to programme the radiographic factors to be used in image acquisition mode. When the acquisition mode is started there may be further updating of the acquisition factors before the ADRC settles on the final factors programme. It is therefore important to ensure the ADRC has stabilised when making QC measurements.

Patient doses, as well as personnel doses, from dynamic imaging are amongst the highest radiation doses found in modern medical practice [4], particularly with respect to entrance surface (skin). Fluoroscopy dominates most procedures in terms of time, whereas in terms of dose, acquisition can account for over half of the total accumulated patient dose [5, 6]. Average dose rates vary between international regions based on prevailing guidance, recommended manufacturer's settings, training, expectations of operators, and to some extent the medical physics community. Nonetheless, there are several reports of tissue reactions or deterministic effects from radiation due to interventional procedures resulting in transient and permanent skin damage [7]. The majority of these are from cardiac [8–10], particularly electrophysiology procedures [11], due to the extended screening (fluoroscopy) times. Stochastic effects on human tissue should also be of concern to minimise radiation-induced cancer and to comply with the 'as low as reasonably practicable' (ALARP) concept [12]. This is of most importance for younger patients whose cells are still differentiating [13]. One of the most significant changes in dynamic imaging performance leading to an increase in the dose is variation of frame rates, which can vary substantially between different modes, and programme, i.e. 0.5 frames per second (fps) for neurological applications and as high as 30 fps for paediatric cardiac applications, where the increased heart rate can cause significant temporal blurring unless high frame rates are used.

X-ray detectors with different coverage areas are available and the selectable field of view (FOV) is matched to the clinical application. For example, a dynamic imaging system in cardiology may have a relatively small (square if FP) image detector with only three FOVs, whereas an interventional vascular system may have large rectangular field coverage with several more FOVs.

References

[1] Worrall M *et al* 2019 IPEM topical report: an evidence and risk assessment based analysis of the efficacy of quality assurance tests on fluoroscopy units-part I: dosimetry and safety *Phys. Med. Biol.* **64** 195011

[2] NEMA 2018 X-ray equipment for interventional procedures user quality control mode *NEMA Standards Publication* XR 27-2013 (R2018) Rosslyn, VA, USA

[3] Hiles P A and Starritt H C 1996 Measurement of the performance characteristics of diagnostic x-ray systems used in medicine: x-ray image intensifier television systems *IPEM Report* 32, part 2 IPEM, York, UK

[4] D'Ercole L, Thyrion F, Bocchiola M, Mantovani L and Klersy C 2012 Proposed local diagnostic reference levels in angiography and interventional neuroradiology and a preliminary analysis according to the complexity of the procedures *Phys. Med.* **28** 61–70

[5] Pitton M, Kloeckner R, Schneider J, Ruckes C, Bersch A and Duber C 2012 Radiation exposure in vascular angiographic procedures *J. Vasc. Interv. Radiol* **23** 1487–95

[6] Davies A G, Cowen A R, Kengyelics S M, Moore J, Pepper C, Cowan C and Sivanathan M U 2006 X-ray dose reduction in fluoroscopically guided electrophysiology procedures *Pacing Clin. Electrophysiol.* **29** 262–71

[7] Vano E, Fernandez J M, Sanchez R M, Martinez D, Lopez Ibor L, Gil A and Serna-Candel C 2013 Patient radiation dose management in the follow-up of potential skin injuries in neuroradiology *Am. J. Neuroradiol.* **34** 277–82

[8] Wagner L 2007 Radiation injury is a potentially serious complication to fluoroscopically-guided complex interventions *Biomed. Imaging Interv. J.* **3** e22

[9] Vlietstra R E, Wagner L K, Koenig T and Mettler F 2004 Radiation burns as a severe complication of fluoroscopically guided cardiological interventions *J. Interv. Cardiol.* **17** 131–42

[10] Balter S 2001 A new tool for benchmarking cardiovascular fluoroscopes *Radiat. Prot. Dosimetry* **94** 161–6

[11] Lickfett L *et al* 2004 Radiation exposure during catheter ablation of atrial fibrillation *Circulation* **110** 3003–11

[12] Department of Health 2000 *The Ionising Radiation (Medical Exposure) Regulations 2000 (Together With Notes on Good Practice)* (London, UK) https://www.legislation.gov.uk/uksi/2000/1059/made

[13] Hall E J 2009 Radiation biology for pediatric radiologists *Pediatr. Radiol.* **39** S57–64

Chapter 2

Dynamic imaging systems

2.1 Overview

The following is a brief description of the main components of a dynamic imaging system, for more detailed information the reader should consult a reference book such as Webb [1], Farr [2], or Dance [3] on the physics of medical imaging or Balter [4] on interventional fluoroscopy physics, technology, and safety.

2.1.1 Types of systems

Fixed tube-detector systems with tilting tables are generally being replaced by more versatile C-arm systems capable of imaging from a wide range of projection angles. These can be mobile systems with a small yoke for image guided manipulation of extremities (so called mini C-arms) or full-size C-arms used as an adjunct to general surgery or ubiquitous in minimal invasive surgery or coronary angiography. Consequently, use of these devices by medical specialists outside the radiology or cardiology department is increasing. This includes orthopaedic, urology, gastroenterology, and vascular surgery [5].

With an increasing range of available medical applications and accompanying procedure complexity, and increasing pressure for manufacturers to provide for improved image quality with lower doses from these systems, there is a requirement for more versatile equipment capable of imaging a wide range of dynamic processes. Consequently, this has led to developments in virtually every component of the imaging chain. Most manufacturers now produce a limited range of base systems with greater flexibility that can be tailored to a broad range of applications. This means that a dynamic imaging system is purchased as a complete system, preconfigured to perform a specific range of procedures, e.g. angiography, cardiology, or neurology, and all containing a common set of components. Modern equipment also includes a number of patient dose saving features (as per International Electrotechnical Commission (IEC) requirements), from displaying the last acquired

doi:10.1088/978-0-7503-3819-6ch2

image, to radiation-free positioning of patient or collimators. This is complemented by the system displaying and storing various dose metrics.

2.1.2 X-ray generator

This basic component of any x-ray imaging system controls the tube voltage, tube current, and exposure duration (pulse width, duration, and rate). Specifically for modern dynamic imaging systems, the generation of x-rays must now include the capability for rapid switching, high power, and long duration x-ray production. Furthermore, in order to optimise patient radiation dose, the feedback mechanism between the x-ray generator and image detector has increased in sophistication and now can include real-time spectral beam adjustment. Highly reproducible x-ray production is essential for imaging systems equipped with DSA because differences in tube voltage between mask and contrast images can cause subtraction artefacts.

2.1.3 X-ray tube assembly

The assembly includes the radiation source, beam filters (static and dynamic), collimators (rectangular and/or iris), and semi-transparent filters (to compensate for extreme contrast differences in the image). X-ray filters (usually copper) are often included as a means of controlling patient (skin) dose while holding image quality at an acceptable level. The collimators are motorised, which allows the collimated x-ray beam to change size in response to adjustment of the SID or when the FOV is changed. Modern systems can include a dose saving feature where the display indicates the position of the collimators and adjustments can be made without the use of radiation ('virtual collimation').

2.1.4 Patient table/couch

For dedicated dynamic x-ray rooms the patient table/couch is an integral part of the equipment, allowing adjustment of the longitudinal, lateral, and vertical positioning of the patient. The table is often cantilevered to allow continuous, unobstructed rotation of the C-arm around the patient during procedures. For some specific applications the table can also be rotated or tilted. It can even be equipped with a motor-driven stepping mechanism for peripheral examination techniques. Any accompanying support mattress can attenuate the x-ray beam and therefore affects patient dose and so should be considered as part of the system when conducting dose measurements. Surgical and other table types which are not made for x-ray purposes can also be used, particularly with mobile C-arms, and should be kept in mind when testing these systems. One of the newest innovations is the incorporation of surgical tables that can break to facilitate anatomical access and dynamic imaging simultaneously: it is, however, in its infancy and therefore beyond the scope of this book.

2.1.5 Anti-scatter grid

The grid is mounted between the patient and detector to reduce the scatter contribution reaching the detector. It should (although may not on some) be possible to remove the grid to reduce patient dose in procedures where low scatter levels are anticipated, such as in paediatric imaging.

2.1.6 Image detector

The image detector must be capable of handling both low dose rate fluoroscopy images and high dose rate acquisitions, achieved by changing detector gain. FP detectors have largely replaced IITV detectors, with the exception that IITV components are still often used in mobile C-arm systems. This has led to more compact designs with increased image processing capabilities, including the possibility of more advanced imaging applications such as 3D or volumetric acquisitions. Some systems permit independent movement of the detector relative to the x-ray tube to provide a variable SID.

2.1.7 Image display

The live image is displayed in real time during a fluoroscopy run, on termination of the run the last image in the series is displayed on the monitor, this is termed last image hold (LIH) Under acquisition, the run is continuously cycled on the monitor and generally sent to PACS for later review. The display also allows selection and adjustment of the mask in subtraction mode. Depending on the application, the system can be equipped with a number of light emitting diode (LED) monitors, or one large user-configurable LED monitor, displaying not only live and stored images, but equipment position information, x-ray generator settings, dose applied, patient monitoring data, and images from other modalities, e.g. ultrasound or optical coherent tomography (OCT). In-room displays can be ceiling mounted and moved, rotated and height adjusted, swivelled and tilted. Some older systems may still have a number of liquid crystal display or even cathode ray tube monitors which display the same information.

2.1.8 Exposure control

The operator can initiate and terminate the x-ray exposure via a footswitch or handswitch. These can include multiple buttons for different exposure functions (fluoroscopy and acquisition modes). It is important to prevent unauthorised or inadvertent use of such controls. In particular, footswitches can be a trip hazard or equipment can be driven into them. This may be heightened by the availability of wireless footswitches which can be easily moved around a room. Some systems provide a useful 'radiation block' control to help prevent accidental exposures.

2.1.9 System control console

System controls can be separated into control modules for equipment movement, x-ray collimation and filtering, dose modes and radiation blocking, and image acquisition, processing, and archiving. Duplicate functions can exist on separate consoles which can be mounted at table-side, on a trolley, and in a separate control room. The system control also includes selection of an appropriate anatomical programme to provide suitable fluoroscopy and acquisition modes. This sets the acquisition and image processing parameters for the imaging task as well as image presentation settings.

2.1.10 Equipment geometry

The x-ray tube assembly and image detector movement are linked. Older static equipment tends to orientate the fixed tube–detector system with the x-ray tube either above or below the couch, termed over- or under-couch, respectively. Most mobile systems and modern static equipment tend to have the tube and detector mounted on a C-arm, a more versatile solution, which is capable of a wide range of rotational movements permitting various cranial/caudal and oblique (right anterior oblique (RAO)/left anterior oblique (LAO)) projections. The C-arm rotates around the centre of rotation, i.e. the isocentre. If an organ is at the isocentre, then its position in the image is constant as the angulation of the C-arm changes. This allows that organ to be seen from different image projections. Static C-arm systems can be floor or ceiling mounted. Biplane systems consist of two C-arms, oriented at 90° to each other, which can be independently positioned around the patient for simultaneous digital acquisitions during a single contrast injection. Mobile systems generally consist of two moveable components, a C-arm mounted on a base unit containing the x-ray generator and a separate display and control system. In some applications the C-arm can be continuously rotated during image acquisition and the data thus obtained used to reconstruct 3D or volume images of the body, a process sometimes referred to as cone beam computed tomography (CT), C-arm CT, or angiographic CT.

2.1.11 Picture archiving and communication system (PACS)

Data transfer, archiving, and storage for modern imaging systems has presented various challenges, such as dealing with extended video sequences and large volumes of acquisition data. Consequently, depending on the compression process, an image retrieved from a PACS system may have reduced image quality compared with the image seen during acquisition [6].

2.2 Automatic dose rate control (ADRC)

There is evidence of a wide variation in doses to patients undergoing similar dynamic imaging procedures at different hospitals [7]. Whilst some of the variation will arise from differences in practice and procedure complexity, there is evidence that wide variation in the initial imaging equipment set up adds substantially to these differences [8]. For almost all dynamic imaging scenarios, modern equipment operates in a mode whereby tube voltage, tube current, and x-ray pulse rate and duration (hereafter referred to as radiographic factors) are determined by an active negative feedback loop between the image detector and the x-ray generator. This feedback loop is referred to as the ADRC mechanism and has a major impact on patient dose and image quality. Consequently, the ADRC should form a crucial component of the commissioning of dynamic imaging systems.

Measurements of the image detector incident air KERMA rate (DAKR) and phantom entrance surface air KERMA rate (ESAKR) [9] provide the physicist with some insight into how a system has been set up, how the system may compare to other dynamic imaging systems used for similar clinical tasks within the service, and whether the current set-up is acceptable or can be improved upon. While comparison between systems can be made using these parameters, one must always remember that the resulting image quality should also be taken into account—and a relevant assessment of image quality between systems is difficult to make. In order to fully characterise the ADRC system performance, it is necessary to measure both the DAKR and ESAKR. The subsequent periodic testing of these dosimetry parameters allows ADRC performance to be tracked over time and can help to identify any changes that may occur. There is generally no simple relationship between DAKR and ESAKR, and this relationship is further weakened in complex systems where tube voltage and spectral filtration changes strongly with patient thickness.

This section provides a detailed overview of the generic ADRC system (figure 2.1); since ADRC designs vary between manufacturers and models, only a generic description is included. Chapter 4 will outline KERMA measurement procedures for DAKR and ESAKR.

Dynamic imaging systems employ sophisticated and flexible ADRC mechanisms that automatically control the radiographic factors, and on some systems this can also include focal spot size, spectral filtration, and target DAKR. This closed loop operating control has the following functions:

1. To automate the selection of radiographic factors required, making the system fast and easy for clinicians and radiographers to use. Manual control

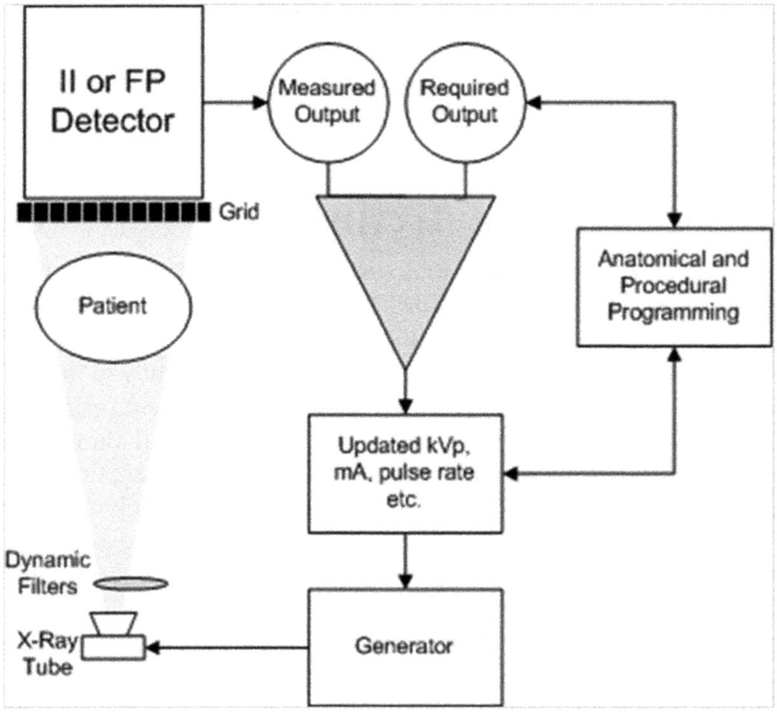

Figure 2.1. Diagram showing a typical ADRC system used in dynamic imaging systems.

of radiographic parameters would be impractical in a busy clinic and operator error could lead to inappropriate radiation dose rates being used.
2. To provide the required level of adequate image quality on a consistent basis. The ADRC should keep image noise at an acceptable level and achieve sufficient contrast. Image quality requirements will vary depending on the clinical task being undertaken.
3. To ensure that the patient dose adheres to local standards or regulations and diagnostic reference levels. The ALARP principle (keep the dose 'as low as reasonably practicable') must be followed.
4. To ensure that the x-ray tube limits are not surpassed, i.e. the tube does not overheat, ensuring a reasonable operating life for the tube and that it will not have to shut down during clinical use.

Although the closed loop operating control is essential for clinical practice, it is something of a black box in nature and detailed descriptions of ADRC operation can be difficult to obtain from manufacturers. In turn, this can make it difficult for the physicist to perform relevant measurements and accurately interpret results. One obvious problem is the lack of direct control over x-ray parameters which greatly complicates tube and generator testing. This can also make it difficult for physicists (even different physicists from the same service) to consistently set up the same programmes for QC testing. An in-depth understanding of how these automated mechanisms control the x-ray beam during image capture definitely helps to address such issues.

2.2.1 Design and function of ADRC mechanisms

ADRC systems sample the output of the II or FP detector and compare this signal to a predetermined target level. If the sampled signal level lies outside some predefined range then the level is corrected by adjusting the settings listed in table 2.1. The point in the imaging chain at which the ADRC samples the detector output can vary between systems [10]. For II based systems, either the light input to the camera can be sampled using a photomultiplier tube or photodiode, or the video signal from the camera itself. For FP based systems the detector output signal is sampled directly. The region of the detector that is sampled by the ADRC will vary from system to

Table 2.1. Possible radiographic settings that can be automatically altered by the ADRC. The top three are always adjusted by the ADRC; the bottom two are only adjusted by the ADRC on some dynamic x-ray systems.

X-ray tube voltage (kVp)
X-ray tube current (mA)
X-ray pulse (frame) duration (ms)
Spectral beam filtration (mm thickness of metal)
Focal spot size (mm)

system, and between specific imaging protocols. The flexibility and ease of use of the sensing region may also vary, depending on system design and sophistication. On some systems the user may have the option of choosing sensing areas of different size, shape, and location for specific clinical tasks, while in other cases only service engineers may have the option to change these areas.

Effective patient thickness is used as the starting point to ascertain the initial radiographic factors set by the x-ray generator. Figures 2.2 through 2.5 show examples of ADRC control curves, demonstrating how settings are selected as a function of patient equivalent thickness in cm of polymethyl methacrylate (PMMA) [11]. On some imaging systems the effective patient thickness is initially set by the clinical programme and/or patient size which were selected by the user. The selected programme will also determine spectral filtration and focal spot settings.

If there was a prior period of fluoroscopy, as is often the case, the effective patient thickness is calculated from data derived from the fluoroscopy sequence. This calculation is based on various settings such as radiographic factors, spectral filtration, SID, and pixel intensity values. This 'effective' patient thickness is then used as the starting point to ascertain the initial radiographic factors set by the x-ray generator, for both fluoroscopy and acquisition runs. It is important to note that for some systems, if the geometric set-up and/or beam attenuating material has been changed, a period of fluoroscopy (usually a few seconds) is required for the new effective patient thickness to be calculated. A useful rule of thumb is to always 'fluoro first' when testing different geometric set-ups or thicknesses of beam attenuation. With regard to acquisition modes (rather than fluoroscopy), all modern systems require a period of fluoroscopy prior to acquisition before setting the image

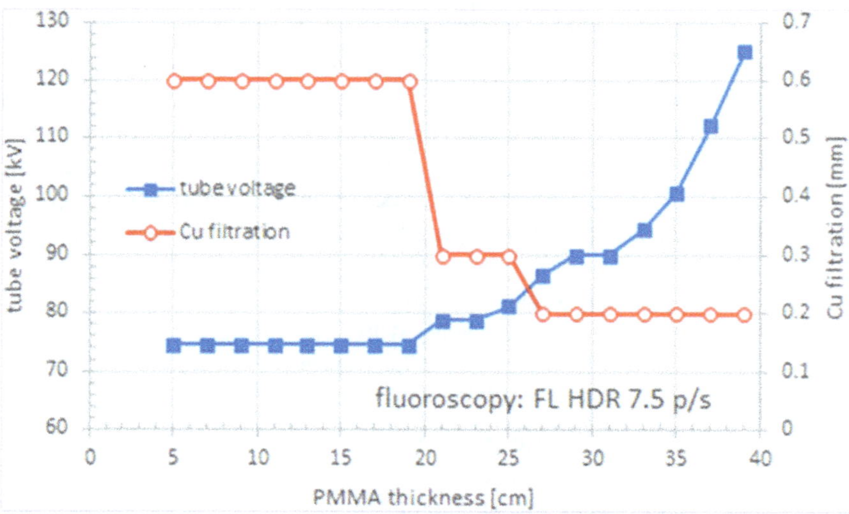

Figure 2.2. Example curves demonstrating the relationship between tube voltage and filtration as a function of PMMA thickness and shows clearly that the filtration in many modern dynamic imaging systems does not remain constant.

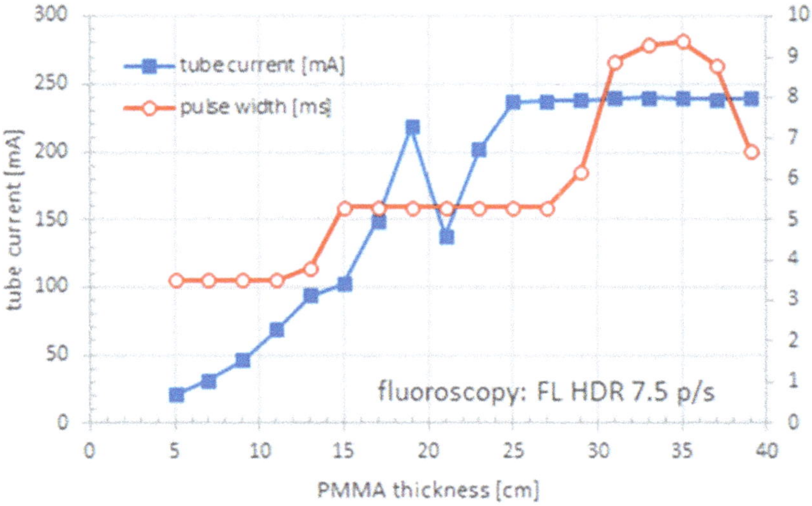

Figure 2.3. Example curves demonstrating the relationship between tube current and pulse width as a function of PMMA thickness and shows that the pulse length is not a constant.

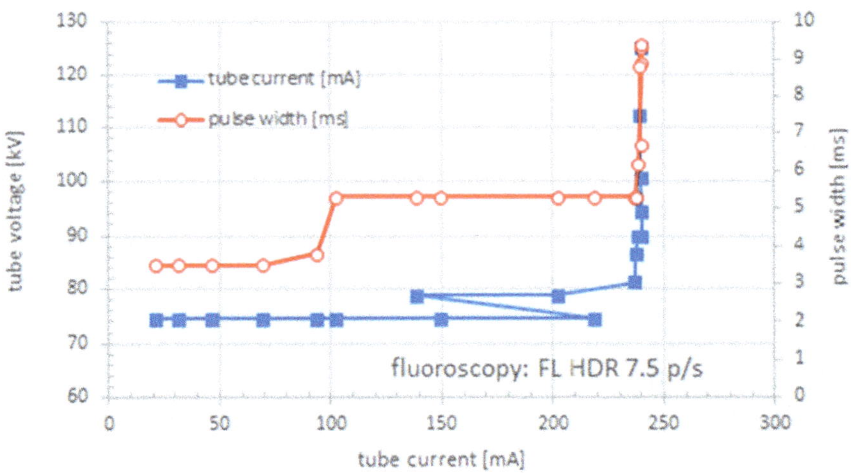

Figure 2.4. Example curves demonstrating the relationship of pulse width in a kVp/mA curve for a cardiac procedure.

acquisition parameters; this was sometimes referred to as fluoroscopy programmed radiography (FPR).

Once an acquisition or fluoroscopy run has begun using these initial radiographic factors, the image detector output frames are sampled. Each user-selectable imaging mode has a programme requested signal level. The difference between the measured and requested signal level is calculated for every image frame and the generator settings updated accordingly for the next image frame. This process is repeated after each frame throughout the run in order to achieve the requested image signal level.

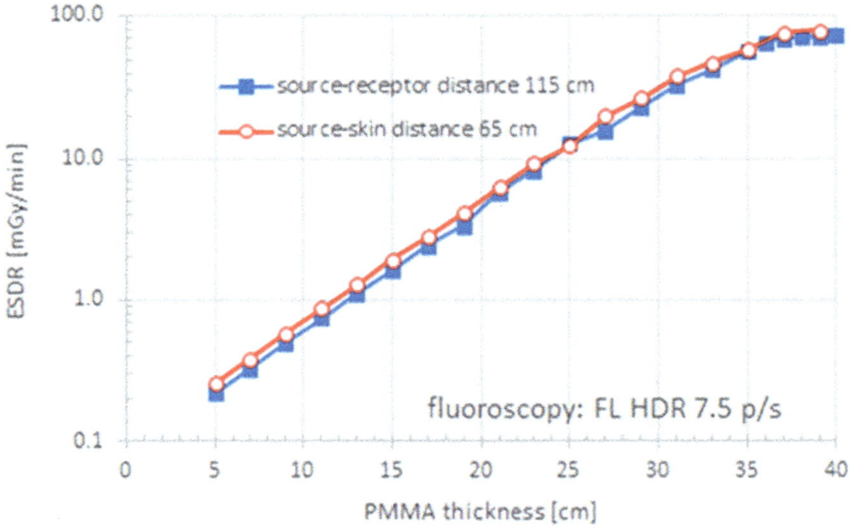

Figure 2.5. Example curves demonstrating the relationship between the entrance surface dose rate (ESAKR) as a function of PMMA thickness.

Some systems begin capture of an image sequence at a relatively fast frame rate, until the requested signal has been met, and then slow down to the required frame rate for that clinical programme for the remainder of the image sequence; it is important to know this before trying to measure dose rate or similar measurements.

The reason for recalculating effective thickness after each fluoroscopy run is to account for changes in geometry and projection (gantry) angle (i.e. rotation and angulation of the C-arm). Some ADRC facilities do not take into consideration the distance between the x-ray source and patient for the effective patient thickness calculation; in these cases the patient table height does not have an impact on operation of the ADRC. Some ADRC designs do not respond to changes in SID or even FOV (although this is unusual).

With reference to table 2.1, the first three rows are referred to as radiographic factors in this report and are generally controlled by ADRC. The latter two are sometimes controlled by ADRC, depending on the x-ray system manufacturer and intended clinical use; if not controlled by the ADRC they are controlled by the selected clinical programme, imaging mode (low dose or normal etc), and sometimes patient size. Materials used for spectral filtration vary, but are generally restricted to copper (Cu), aluminium (Al), or a combination of the two. However, tantalum (Ta) can also be found in a minority of systems. Some systems have ADRC controlled filtration, whereas systems with fixed filtration (for a given imaging mode) do not adjust filtration within an image sequence; the former filtration systems are often referred to as a Seizl filter [10]. Systems with more than one focal spot may have the ADRC programmed to switch to the smaller focal spot size in order to reduce spatial blurring where possible [11].

In DSA the ADRC operation differs slightly from that described here. Some systems utilise a test shot at the start of the DSA run using initial radiographic factors obtained from the previous fluoroscopy sequence. The sampled signal from this image is compared to the requested signal, and radiographic factors are established for the DSA run. In contrast to fluoroscopy, DSA factors are not updated during the acquisition sequence. On older systems a substantial dose can be delivered in the test shot; if possible it may be useful to set a delay such that the test shot dose can be recorded, followed by a meter reset to measure the dose for the main sequence. DSA programmes employ a mask; this is an image from the beginning of the run (i.e. before the contrast has been injected) that is then subtracted from all images in the run to form the subtraction images. The mask image can be changed (the run can be re-masked) retrospectively by the user. DSA often operates at higher dose levels compared to non-subtracted programmes (sometimes referred to as native acquisition), typically at a factor of two greater than native programmes. This is to overcome the increased stochastic noise in the subtracted images. Subtraction of the mask from a contrast image increases the variance of uncorrelated noise in the two images by a factor of two, although any lag present will introduce some correlation for images with only a small temporal separation.

2.2.2 ADRC dose control curves

Settings are adjusted with respect to the patient thickness, which not only depends on patient size but also on the projection angle used for imaging because a steeper angle results in a larger effective patient thickness. Fixed filter systems tend to select tube voltage based on patient thickness, with tube current and frame duration selected based on tube voltage. X-ray systems with a Seizl filter tend to adjust spectral filtration to optimise x-ray beam energy with respect to the patient size [12, 13], i.e. they change both the tube voltage and the filtration together; tube current and x-ray frame duration are selected based on the beam energy (tube voltage and filtration combination) used. Either way, radiographic factors are selected to attain the level of image quality required for the given imaging mode, acquisition (including DSA), or fluoroscopy, and clinical procedure.

Examples of how a system may change radiographic factors with patient thickness are shown in figures 2.2–2.5. The x-ray system was set up using the given amount of PMMA in the posterior–anterior (PA) projection. The anatomical programme chosen was cardiac fluoroscopy, running at 7.5 fps.

Clearly, there is a complex interaction between tube voltage, mA, spectral filtration, and pulse width, and one of the tasks of the QC physicist is to understand the interplay between these parameters as a function of patient equivalent thickness. It is therefore important that the ADRC and associated image quality is assessed under clinically relevant conditions (rather than some dedicated 'physics' type mode)—not doing so can lead to problems/discussion between the manufacturer, the physics department, and the clinicians. Some of these issues will be addressed in the image quality chapter.

2.2.3 Automatic gain control (AGC)

Fluctuations in radiographic factors as the ADRC stabilises are usually not visualised by users at the beginning of an image sequence; this is the influence of automatic gain control (AGC) that operates alongside the ADRC. Image gain is used to adjust the digital pixel values and hence the appearance of an x-ray image. Images with low average signal (brightness), due to insufficient x-ray penetration through the patient, are electronically amplified, which ultimately increases final displayed luminance. Hence, AGC circuits have a different influence on image noise (electronic and quantum) compared to ADRC control of radiographic factors alone (no AGC).

The AGC operates automatically and can be considered to be a subcomponent of the ADRC system. Some gain control systems operate by normalising each image frame to the same target pixel value, for optimal viewing by clinicians depending on the clinical application or mode selected. This pixel value corresponds with the requested image signal referred to in section 2.2.1.

On older systems the x-ray generator response to feedback from the ADRC facility is often slower to reach the new radiographic factors compared to modern systems. Adjustment of the gain applied to the video signal prior to display can be performed on a shorter timescale to allow a useful image to be displayed during the response time. On state-of-the-art systems, the response is effectively instantaneous, however, the first few frames of an image sequence are required before the requested image signal is actually reached.

2.2.4 Selection of radiographic factors

The displayed radiographic factors may vary between different imaging modes and between different manufacturers. For most (but not all) manufacturers, peak tube voltage and peak tube current, as well as the frame pulse length, are all reported for acquisition runs, whereas the frame pulse length is not reported for fluoroscopy runs. The tube current is generally reported differently for fluoroscopy than for acquisition. The reported fluoroscopy value may be referred to as the continuous equivalent tube current [14]; it is the tube current multiplied by the fraction of the frame cycle where irradiation occurs, known as the duty factor (frame rate (in fps) × frame length (seconds)). For example 21 mA continuous equivalent tube current (as reported in fluoroscopy) refers to 200 mA peak tube current (as reported in acquisition) for 15 fps and 7 ms pulse duration.

The characteristics and limitations of the imaging system x-ray tube and generator play an important role in ADRC selection of radiographic factors. Specific power constraints will prohibit the use of certain combinations of radiographic factors, as explained in the remainder of this section. The x-ray tube and generator will have a range of values that are available (for example 40–125 kV and 50–1000 mA). However, certain combinations of factors cannot be used together, for instance high kV, high tube current combinations, and low kV, high tube current combinations; exact combinations will differ between systems. Figure 2.6 shows examples of available kV–mA values for various imaging modes. Grey shading

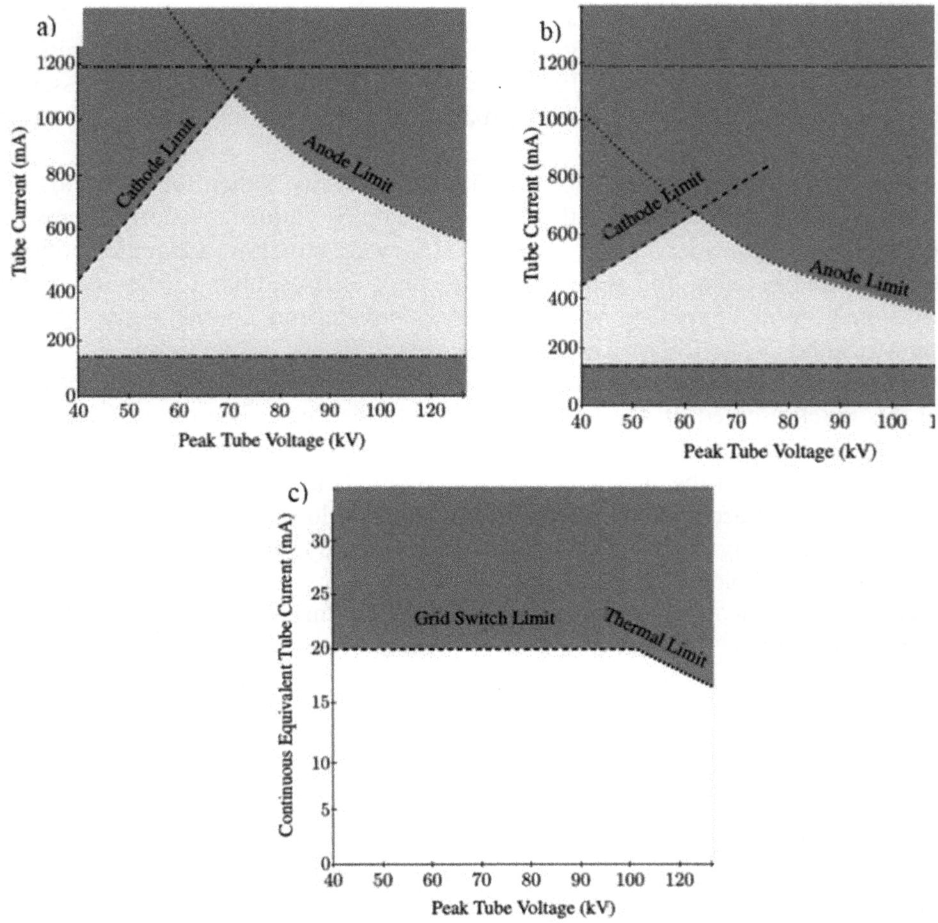

Figure 2.6. (a) Limitations of radiographic factors are shown for acquisition using a large focus; actual values depend on the x-ray tube ratings and generator used. (b) Limitations of radiographic factors are shown an acquisition using a fine focus. (c) Tube limitations are shown for fluoroscopy. In fluoroscopy, some systems use a 'grid switch' to remove ramp and tail edges of x-ray frames in an effort to reduce motion blur and low energy radiation which does not contribute to image quality. To ensure stability of the emitter structure under grid switch conditions some manufacturers limit the maximum x-ray tube current to be used. This creates a flat roof to the open space as shown here.

indicates combinations that are not permissible; all systems are different and these are only examples.

The x-ray tube anode introduces two main limits related to heating of the focal track and the heat capacity and rate of cooling of the anode assembly. Focal track heating is principally an issue in higher x-ray output operating modes, i.e. cardiac acquisition and DSA. This is a thermal limit set to avoid thermal damage of the focal track. The actual numerical values of this limit depend on the x-ray tube type, focal spot size, length of image run, and duty factor. For example, the duty factor may double when switching from cardiac image acquisition ($15\ \text{f s}^{-1} \times 7\ \text{ms} = 0.1$) to neuro DSA mode (2 fps × 125 ms = 0.2), necessitating a lower anode limit. A lower anode limit would increase the grey region in figure 2.6(c) reducing the range of available settings (white space). In addition to the focal track, the anode assembly must not overheat. The specific heat capacity of the anode and its rate of cooling affect this limit.

Heating within the x-ray tube assembly and x-ray generator must also be controlled. This problem is mostly limited to lengthy fluoroscopy procedures and is controlled by imposing a fixed power load ('isowatt') to allow adequate cooling of the x-ray tube housing and generator. The curve looks similar to the anode limit shown in grey in figure 2.6, where actual values depend on the x-ray tube and generator used.

Operation of the x-ray tube filament also has a limitation, namely the cathode, and this is represented on the figures by the cathode limit. Electron emission from the cathode is restricted at low x-ray tube voltage. Actual values of the cathode limit depend on the x-ray tube and focal spot size. A clinician may wish to use the smaller focal spot to increase spatial resolution, but this will lower the anode and cathode limits, thus altering which radiographic factors may be selected as shown in figure 2.6. The choice of a small focal spot size limits the maximum mA, which for large patients would mean increasing the frame duration to a level that would result in motion blur for some applications such as cardiac. The choice of focal spot size is therefore largely dependent on a trade-off between increased motion unsharpness for long frame durations, and increased geometric unsharpness for large focal spot sizes.

2.2.5 Interventional reference point (IRP)

Additionally, manufacturers have to design their ADRC to adhere to the strict national standards implemented by the various countries in which they do business. For example, the Food and Drug Association (FDA, USA) has set a limit of 10 R min^{-1} (88 mGy min^{-1}) in fluoroscopy patient exposure rates [15]. The IEC on the other hand, stipulate that two default fluoroscopy modes within one clinical application be designed such that when a user switches from the lower dose to higher dose mode, the patient dose rate is at most doubled, for reference air KERMA measurements [16].

Both the FDA and the IEC refer to the incident air KERMA (without backscatter). However, the FDA and IEC each define different measurement points, as shown in figure 2.7. The IEC patient entrance reference point for air KERMA is defined 15 cm from the isocentre in the direction of the x-ray tube (for undercouch tube systems); this is more widely known as the interventional reference point (IRP). The FDA measurement point is defined 30 cm in front of the detector entrance surface and is therefore dependent on SID. When the detector is moved the FDA dose point changes and the radiographic factors required to maintain the same limiting patient dose rate also change due to the inverse square law.

ADRC systems are therefore designed to select radiographic factors such that these standards and limits are adhered to. Past UK guidelines [17] stated that

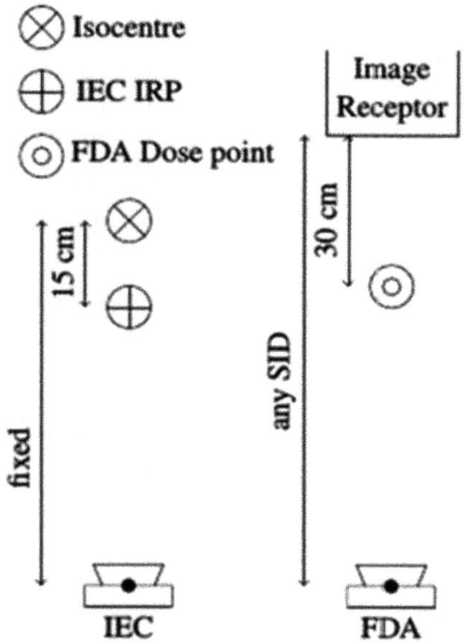

Figure 2.7. Diagrams illustrating the difference between the FDA and the IEC interventional reference points.

remedial action is required where the ESAKR exceeds 50 mGy min^{-1} for 20 cm water on the largest available field of view. The revised guidelines [18] reflect the changes in modern equipment and no longer include these limits. It is now understood that the ADRC is designed with inherent limits for FDA and IEC regulations, and that any issues found with dose rates should be addressed by the relevant medical physics expert (MPE).

The ADRC curves shown in figures 2.2–2.5, as well as the description of ADRC function, highlight the role of effective patient thickness in ADRC operation. It is important to note that this does not simply refer to the range of patient sizes within a given population. During a single procedure, effective patient thickness will vary as projection (i.e. gantry angle) changes. For example, where in cardiac imaging a PA view of the heart typically shows internal system-calculated patient thicknesses of 22–24 cm, the 'spider view' thicknesses can be as large as 40 cm. The spider view is RAO 30–40 degrees, caudal 30–40 degrees, whereas straight PA is near 0 and 0 degrees. Similarly, for neuro x-ray imaging there may be differences of approximately 6 cm between lateral and frontal anatomic projections [14].

2.3 Additional features of dynamic imaging systems

Because dynamic imaging lends itself to a large range of clinical uses in modern medicine, it should not be surprising that there are a correspondingly large number of additional features available in these systems. Some of these are described in the following sections:

2.3.1 Dose reporting systems

Since the early days of fluoroscopy it has been accepted that patient skin doses can be extremely high, with the potential to cause serious injury to the patient's skin. Whilst individual responses to radiation vary significantly, threshold doses for a variety of tissue reactions/deterministic effects have been recognised and published by the ICRP [19]. Many years ago it was recognised that some form of dose mitigation, often guided by automatic prompts from the equipment, is required. For this purpose, to focus the attention of the operator, fluoroscopy systems have had fluoroscopy or 'beam on' timers for many years.

2.3.1.1 Fluoroscopy timer

The fluoroscopy timer and consequent five and ten minute alarms are present on all systems, in compliance with IEC 60601-2-43 [16]. These functions were originally intended to highlight the period of continuous fluoroscopy time to the operator and, in conjunction with last image hold, have led to a reduction in examination 'beam on' times.

The use of the fluoroscopy timer on some modern systems may now in fact be misleading. Some manufacturers of pulsed fluoroscopy equipment continue to use the original 'beam on' definition of fluoroscopy time, so may not hit the 5 min warning despite 5 min of imaging ('pedal time'). Therefore, use of just the timer as an indication of patient dose can lead to inaccuracies. Due to short-duration/high-output pulsing of the beam, the patient exposure from such systems may be more significant than operators realise and so fluoroscopy time is not considered a suitable measurement of patient dose [20].

2.3.1.2 KERMA area product

The current implementation of IEC 60601-2-43 for interventional x-ray systems [22] has supplemented the basic fluoroscopy timer requirement with a more quantitative measure of patient skin dose. This requirement is also included in FDA CFR part 1020.32 [15], although with some variation of implementation. An air ionisation chamber at the exit of the beam collimator is found on nearly all new x-ray equipment and provides an effective way of directly measuring air KERMA area product (KAP). KAP provides a means of estimating the energy imparted to patients which can be used to quantify the risk of radiation induced carcinogenesis arising from x-ray exposures [21].

Whilst the KAP value does quantify a dose value associated with the patient, the air KERMA at the skin surface is still uncertain unless knowledge of the field size and projection angles is known. Further uncertainty is added from the KAP meter itself which will have a quoted accuracy of not better than 35% [22], although routine QA results would suggest more consistent and accurate results are achievable. Should a true skin dose be required then a backscatter factor for the area irradiated is required, which may vary between 1.3 and 1.5 at diagnostic beam qualities [23], along with the ratio of mass energy absorption coefficients to convert air KERMA to absorbed dose. However, with some conservative judgement, KAP trigger levels can be used in patient dose management [24].

Some manufacturers do not include direct KAP measurement devices in their products and instead use internal look-up tables to generate a calculated KAP value for all normal radiation outputs [25]. The error associated with this method is determined by output stability and collimator positional error. The error will be of a similar order of magnitude to a conventional air ionisation chamber type KAP meter.

2.3.1.3 Peak skin dose (rate)

The current IEC and FDA standards for interventional x-ray equipment build on the principle of KAP measurements to provide users with two derivative values corrected for radiation field size. Both standards require reporting of the cumulative air KERMA and air KERMA rate at a defined reference point to represent the entrance surface of the patient (see figure 2.7). The uncertainty allowed in this measurement, 35% according to the FDA [15], is increased over that of the KAP only measurement to reflect errors in field size in the calculation. Whilst the KERMA measurements are a step-wise improvement on KAP, they are limited by the standardised reference points which do not fully account for patient size, table position, movement, or variations in imaging geometry during the procedure.

All dose is assumed to be deposited at a single point on the patient skin and does not change throughout the procedure. While this is an estimate of patient skin dose that can be seen by the operator, the accumulated air KERMA reported will overestimate the dose if the patient is further away than the reference point, and underestimate the radiation dose at steep angles laterally where the patient is closer. This method still does not apply a backscatter correction or ratio of mass energy absorption coefficients to the value reported. Therefore this parameter can currently only be considered as an approximate estimate of peak skin dose.

2.3.1.4 Skin dose mapping

The most recent iteration of this line of skin dose estimate takes into account patient shape and projection angle to calculate a more realistic cumulative skin dose [26]. This advanced built-in system will map the doses generated for IEC and FDA compliance onto a three-dimensional patient model. This technology is not standardised at the time of writing, with proprietary implementations by most of the major manufacturers in interventional radiology, which provide active dose mapping during procedures.

There are also third-party software applications which will produce similar results retrospectively from Digital Imaging and Communications in Medicine (DICOM) Radiation Dose Structured Reports (RSDR) (e.g. OpenSkin for OpenREM). All the active dose mapping systems use geometrical information about the angle of projection, field size, and previous dose delivered to the skin to calculate the dose distribution in false colour on a voxelised phantom patient. The skin of the phantom is often unwrapped to allow clearer visualisation. The position of peak skin dose is normally indicated and the current field of view overlaid so that alternative projections can be identified [27].

The dose mapping options available commercially are mostly based on an elliptic cylinder body shape but Rana *et al* [28] have used a 3D humanoid model in the Canon (formerly Toshiba) Dose Tracking System (DTS), in which doses are projected on to a user selectable body shape scaled for height, weight, and sex. In a later version [28] the model has been modified based on AP and lateral projections of the patient taken prior to the procedure. The dose data for the model are based on independent look-up tables of dose per mAs calibrated in an appropriate scatter environment to allow backscatter corrected mapping onto the patient surface. The authors claim an accuracy of −3, +7% in reproducing the dose compared to using a 6cc ionisation chamber on the patient surface.

As export of dose data is becoming standardised, many manufacturers have now implemented dose mapping in their dose tracking software as part of their PACS data including Sectra (DoseTrack), GE Healthcare (Dosewatch), Bayer (Radimetrics), Siemens (Syngo Workflow Dose Management module), and Qaelum (DOSE). These data are not only for offline review; it is also useful to the operator to monitor how peak skin dose varies with projection as the procedure progresses.

The most accurate skin dose mapping is carried out using calibrated radiochromic film wrapped around the patient [23] and is considered by many to remain the gold standard in identifying peak absorbed dose. The dosimetry in this method has significantly lower uncertainty associated with it (−12.8%, +10.0%) compared to indirect methods. The errors are primarily due to calibration uncertainty and the energy dependence of the film used. There can be some additional uncertainty in ascribing the dose location to the patient's skin but this applies to all dose mapping systems. The process of calibrating radiochromic film is well established in radiotherapy physics and translates well to skin dose measurement in lengthy cardiology and interventional radiology cases. However, due to the cost of the film it is difficult to justify this routinely when other methods are available.

2.3.2 Advanced digital subtraction angiography (DSA)/road mapping

DSA is a technique used to remove overlying anatomical structures while imaging the vascular system. In the most basic mode, a pre-contrast mask image is obtained of the region of interest which is then subtracted from subsequent images (i.e. containing the contrast). Anatomical structures that occur in both images are removed from the subtracted image, while the contrast in the vasculature remains and is easier to see. Image processing is frequently applied because noise in the two images adds during the subtraction step. Frame averaging and smoothing algorithms are frequently used to minimise the noise in the mask before storing. In addition, the DSA run image may also use frame averaging or smoothing with the consequence that the actual frame rate may be different to the anatomical programme selected. DSA removes anatomical structure from the image and forms one of the most important techniques in the diagnosis of defects in the vasculature. Mis-registration artefacts are a common problem in DSA and arise due to movement of the anatomy between the mask acquisition and later contrast acquisitions. Pixel shifting techniques are used to correct for movement lateral to the image plane and these can be very advanced. The Clarity processing developed by Philips allows automatic submillimetre shifting of local image regions. Rotation can be corrected for in some of the newest equipment from Siemens. However, none of the authors have any experience of this.

Road mapping is useful for the placement of catheters and wires in complex and small vasculature. Road mapping is similar to DSA in that a DSA sequence is performed. The frame with maximum contrast opacity is identified and used as a road map mask. This mask is then subtracted from a live screening run to produce real-time subtracted fluoroscopic image overlaid on a static image of the vasculature. Therefore, catheters are visualised over an image of the vasculature.

2.3.3 3D rotational angiography (3DRA) and cone beam computed tomography (CBCT)

In this mode, a series of images are acquired as the C-arm rotates through at least 180 degrees around the patient and covering a large anatomic region of interest. The acquired volumetric data set can then be reconstructed in the axial, coronal, or sagittal planes or as a rotatable 3D image. For C-arm CBCT systems, current detector arrays are 40×30 cm^2, allowing $25 \times 25 \times 18$ cm^3 volumetric datasets to be generated in a single rotation of the source and detector [29]. Cone beam CT has several disadvantages compared to fan beam CT, including the time delay in viewing the image (CBCT acquisition time 5–20 s plus further 60 s for reconstruction) and the increased scattered radiation (due to the wider x-ray beam collimation) leading to lower image quality. CBCT can be used in conjunction with contrast media to produce vasculature enhanced images as already mentioned, with the advantage that with one rotational acquisition several projections of the vascular region are obtained with one injection, a spatial visualisation of the course of the vessels is possible, and a rotational 3D image can be generated. With rotational angiography it is essential that the volume of interest should be positioned at the isocentre of the C-arm, otherwise it may move out of the image area in some projections.

2.3.4 NEMA: user quality control mode

Dynamic imaging has evolved from hardware based open-loop control to software-based feedback-stabilised control, which has been implemented differently by different manufacturers; thus making it difficult to provide a standardised list of consistent QC tests. In addition, digital technologies have decoupled the link between input air KERMA and pixel value; allowing a much greater parameter space from which clinically acceptable images can be generated. It is therefore difficult to ensure consistency of equipment performance, in particular between similar systems from different manufacturers. User control has also evolved to the point where single protocol selections now commonly control/select many different underlying parameters (of which only a few are typically visible to the operator).

User QC mode (UQCM) is a NEMA standard [2] that enables a QC measurement mode via a password. The standard was initially applicable for fixed interventional equipment only, but has since been extended for mobile interventional equipment via an additional amendment. UQCM provides one or more QC user interfaces that will allow the user to perform the following tests through selection of values, either by manual control, or by preset combination values, for tube voltage, current, exposure time, spectral filtration, and focal spot size. While x-ray tube protection mechanisms will remain active, the detector will be vulnerable to excessive radiation exposure and therefore the onus is on the tester to protect the detector in this mode.

1. Half-value layer.
2. Dose reproducibility.
3. Tube current linearity.
4. Tube voltage, tube current, pulse width accuracy.
5. Cumulative air KERMA and KERMA area product (KAP) accuracy.
6. X-ray tube output measurement.

Furthermore, the user will have access to the following applications:

1. Electronic documentation of the system configuration such that the system protocol settings behind the Exam Protocol Selection Buttons (EPSBs) (as defined in the NEMA document) can be exported, e.g. via a memory stick, in a format that can be read in a spreadsheet. Parameters influencing radiation dose (therefore image quality to some extent) should be included: beam filtration, focal spot size, and target kV, mAs, and detector entrance dose values. Differences between the factory default set and locally set parameters should be flagged as this simplifies the review and clinical audit processes.
2. The ability to export images for both presentation and processing purposes and to facilitate both image quality visual tests and quantitative testing.
3. A means to access the radiation dose structured report (RDSR)
4. The ability to change the calibration of the cumulative air KERMA and KAP values on RDSRs.

At the time of writing there was little information from the vendors as to the current implementation status of this mode. It is likely that users (e.g. QC physicists) will have to undergo some training before given access to this mode.

2.4 Introduction to QC of dynamic imaging systems

2.4.1 Preparation for testing

The ADRC controlled nature of the dynamic imaging system, together with the range of system types which are available for different clinical applications, can make the medical physicist's job challenging. The closed loop operating control of radiographic factors can make it difficult to perform measurements, or to accurately interpret results. Hence the need to think ahead when performing acceptance or QC tests on these x-ray systems, ensuring that the testing regime is relevant to the clinical application at hand. The physicist may need to schedule more time than anticipated, particularly for the first set of tests.

Most dynamic imaging systems do not allow for the so-called three button control of radiographic factors, and factors can only be controlled via the internal ADRC, even when it is possible to force a particular tube voltage. Generally, it will not be possible to set a specific set of factors (e.g. kV, mA, and ms) by introducing a certain phantom thickness (and perhaps composition). It will be possible to adjust thickness to obtain some tube voltage but the mA and ms will be set by the system (and will depend on the ADRC mode). The thickness required to do so will vary between different imaging protocols which utilise differing ADRC control curves. Some imaging systems have ADRC, which not only adjusts the radiographic factors but also the spectral filtration and focal spot size in response to patient thickness, as discussed in section 2.2. If the phantom thickness is adjusted, the filtration or focus may also change. Imaging of large patients at steep angles leads to high water equivalent thicknesses—this can be over 40 cm for a cardiac spider view. To accurately represent clinical practice you may need to use thick phantoms, depending on the clinical application. The department radiographers can tell you how steep the angles used are, as can DICOM headers of patient image sequences (e.g. DICOM tag 0018,1510 Positioner Primary Angle: 30).

When testing these systems the foot pedal must be held down for long enough for the ADRC to stabilise; otherwise the factors which you record will not accurately represent the dose rate at which the system settles for use. However, the image sequence shown as the pedal is depressed may appear to be consistent from the first or second frame. This is because of an internal image gain mechanism which is applied to each image frame in real time to account for the image quality not being adequate, i.e. makes it look as though the radiographic factors were sufficient from the start. Some systems require the 'fluoro first' rule: change phantom thickness or geometry; depress the fluoroscopy pedal for a few seconds prior to a DSA or acquisition image sequence. The fluoroscopy image sequence should then be ignored in terms of measurements. This allows for the ADRC to re-calibrate for the new x-ray set-up.

2.4.2 Advice on when, what, and how to test

If during QC testing, the ADRC responds differently to the same geometric set-up, phantom type, and thickness and imaging mode (whether fluoroscopy or acquisition), as set for/at the previous test, then this is an indication that the underlying dose control curves or target dose levels may have been changed for that mode.

Ideally, the programmed parameters for the mode in question should be visible to the operator and can be checked or confirmed by visual inspection. In the future, for systems where the NEMA UQCM is available (see section 2.3.4), the first step in QC would be to export the ADRC settings to a spreadsheet. Then the programmes/modes can be examined for changes in parameters/settings. Where this becomes problematic is when all discernible parameters and/or settings remain unchanged but there are differences in x-ray settings which are only accessible to high level service engineers. The user should be notified of such changes and the department should proceed with clinical work in the new adjusted mode only after testing and the dose levels (and associated image quality) are found to be acceptable [30].

Ideally, the user will be notified in advance that a manufacturer applications specialist or engineer will be adjusting the system. Section 2.4.3 discusses the multi-disciplinary team working concept which can help increase communications between everyone who comes into contact with the imaging system in question. Prompt notification will allow for the appropriate amount of time to be scheduled in the department for testing to be completed, (between the change taking place and the first clinical use after the change has taken place). It may be necessary to re-measure the kV–mA curve to determine whether or not the ADRC control curves of a given mode have been changed. This can most easily be accomplished by adding increasingly larger amounts of PMMA between the detector and tube and recording the tube voltage and tube current for each thickness, for fluoroscopy and acquisition modes. Note that this can become more complicated if spectral filter, focal spot, and/or variable pulse rates are changed by the system for the programme under test.

Imaging modes often have a frame rate in their name e.g. 'Left Coronary 15 fps' or 'Neuro DSA 2 fps'; it should not be assumed that this frame rate is constant. When a common clinical application is performed manufacturers may programme the imaging mode to adjust frame rates in the middle of the image sequence as per the known clinical method. For example, in neuro imaging the venous phase has a slow movement of contrast medium whereas the arterial phase is fast, so frame rates may be programmed to change accordingly. However, within one DSA image sequence, radiographic factors are generally fixed. This may impact on dose measurement, depending whether dose rate or accumulated dose is being displayed on the dosimeter.

Some manufacturers also allow for the set-up of a physics imaging mode specifically for QA testing [21]. This would ideally allow for both control of settings in table 2.1 and the accessibility of unprocessed images with a linear response to DAKR. 'Linear' in this context means that the pixel value is linear with the DAKR without backscatter (see chapter 7 for image quality assessments). At the time of publication this was not routinely provided; physicists who wish access to such a mode should request this via the application specialist, the service engineer or perhaps even the design/system engineers (generally this is difficult to access). This is likely to change with the introduction of the UQCM (section 2.3.8).

2.4.3 Multi-disciplinary team (MDT) working

It is important to understand that the shift in technology that has occurred in the last few decades has been far reaching in dynamic imaging systems. In particular, the shift to full software control has allowed manufacturers to substantially increase the ability to tailor image quality and dose to customers' clinical requirements. The disadvantage of this technological advance is that there can be hundreds of settings associated with each imaging examination protocol; in most cases visible only to service engineers. These settings range from dose control curves (which operate the ADRC) to image enhancement algorithms; differences between imaging protocols may be subtle but there is potential for many differences to be missed.

Fitting the testing regime to the clinical application is essential to avoid spending time on unnecessary tests. Therefore, before starting any acceptance or commissioning measurements, it is recommended that the physicist completes two tasks. First, get to know the system before the commissioning baselines are measured. Spending time examining a system before commissioning can save considerable time later on. For example, some manufacturers use one kV–mA curve for a number of anatomical programmes. Second, and just as important, the physicist should speak to the staff who will use the system: knowledge of what the system will be used for and an understanding of what programmes should be on the system will give some idea of how it should be set up. Working as part of a multi-disciplinary team (MDT) is the best way to achieve this. It should also not be assumed that the default manufacturer programmes are optimised for local practice—they may be adequate but some adjustment may be needed to account for local service requirements. An MDT will help assure that *all* involved have communicated the needs of the local service as well as potential upcoming changes to prepare for. Medical physics teams are moving further away from working in isolation and more towards working in MDTs to assure x-ray systems are optimised not only for ALARP settings but also for particular clinical procedures which are performed locally.

The first test of a dynamic imaging system is involved and will take considerable time; interventional, cardiology, and other complex systems may take a number of days and time should be agreed for this. Clearly less complex systems take less time. While ideally, dose rate and image quality information for all protocols, field sizes, and patient sizes should be obtained, it is frequently impossible to justify the time required to do so. As a bare minimum the following should be obtained:

1. Dose rates for all FOVs of the most commonly used anatomical programme.
2. Dose rates for most common programmes for one FOV.
3. Dose rates for different patient sizes for one FOV and anatomical programme.

In particular with the more complex systems, there are a great many subtle differences that are not immediately obvious, which clearly makes testing difficult and subsequent investigation problematic. For example, for the same anatomical programme a smaller focal spot may be required for a paediatric mode than for an adult mode. Most (certainly all modern) x-ray tubes and generators have different intrinsic limits associated with differing focal spot sizes, and this will be seen in the different radiographic factors selected by the ADRC. Furthermore, most manufacturers set different intrinsic limits for the combinations of image frame rates and x-ray pulse durations (called the duty factor, see section 2.2.4 for more detail). Therefore it should not be assumed that just because two anatomical programmes appear to operate in the same way, they are the same; deviation may occur for different FOVs.

As another example, neurological DSA (requiring a small frame rate and long frame duration) would have a lower anode limit than cardiac acquisition (requiring a larger frame rate but short frame duration) and therefore the ADRC would not allow the x-ray tube current to be set as high as in cardiac acquisition. For each DSA or acquisition imaging mode, there are typically three fluoroscopy imaging modes, representing three different dose rates no higher than the 8.8 cGy/min maximum FDA legal limit [15]. The tableside controls allow easy switching between these modes. Note that the modes assigned to these buttons/controls can be reprogrammed (perhaps under service control). These fluoroscopy imaging protocols tend to be the same within a clinical application group, although this is not always the case.

To further complicate matters this is not generally made clear by the labelling and therefore most fluoroscopy imaging protocols should still be tested at least during commissioning or acceptance testing to ascertain under which clinical application groups, they operate differently. It should not be assumed for example that for all vascular or cardiac imaging the three fluoroscopy imaging protocols are the same. Calling up a cardiac acquisition programme means the fluoroscopy buttons reflect cardiac settings, while calling up a vascular (neuro) DSA acquisition programme means the fluoroscopy buttons reflect neuro settings (with different recursive filtering, target DAKR, etc, internally programmed). In the interest of optimisation, manufacturers are increasing the number of different fluoroscopy imaging programmes available to users that will suit a given clinical procedure and/or patient size. Working with an MDT may help keep communication between different departments as well as the manufacturer staff; this is relevant because there may be a pending visit from an applications specialist to adjust the programmed settings for optimisation purposes (see section 2.4.4). That being the case it would be more time-efficient to perform commissioning after the applications visit, or complete a smaller routine test after the applications visit.

The authors are aware of the difficulty in designing and performing QC on such complex systems within the often severely limited time available for testing. However, software control can cause changes in unpredictable ways and the only way to mitigate against this is a good set of baseline measurements to be able to find changes to often untested imaging modes.

2.4.4 Advice on quality control issues

During routine QC testing, if the ADRC is seen to respond differently to the same geometric set-up and phantom thickness as used for previous tests, then the manufacturer may have adjusted the system such that the dose control curves changed for that mode. Internal imaging mode settings can only be changed by high level service engineers or other specified manufacturer employees. When a change has been made the department should have been notified in advance, and should proceed with clinical work in the new mode only after testing and confirmation of acceptable dose levels. There have been a number of cases where database values holding the system parameters have been altered after standard software upgrades or the system has been returned to factory default settings after a service and the local settings need to be re-implemented.

Imaging protocols which utilise road mapping (see section 2.3.2) may be very complex. Different manufacturers design road mapping tools differently and, unless there is a clear understanding of how these tools are used by clinicians, it is not easy to obtain a clinically meaningful measurement of radiation dose. Relatively high patient dose rates can result from such tools; hence the need to assure that any measurements being reported actually represent clinical practice.

2.4.5 Manufacturer applications specialists/trainers

Manufacturer applications specialists generally tend to visit after acceptance and commissioning has been completed. This may result in different set-ups such that the baselines are no longer relevant, making it impossible to identify changes in system performance and forcing a re-measurement of baselines. Two options are available to minimise this problem: perform commissioning after the applications visit, or complete a smaller routine test after the applications visit. Either way, there is a requirement for greater access to equipment as well as a higher workload for medical physics departments than there was in the past.

References

[1] Flower M 2012 *Webb's Physics of Medical Imaging* 2nd edn (Boca Raton, FL: Taylor and Francis)

[2] NEMA 2018 X-ray equipment for interventional procedures user quality control mode *NEMA Standards Publication XR 27-2013 (R2018)* (Rosslyn, VA)

[3] Dance D R, Christofides S, Mclean I D and Ng K H 2013 *Diagnostic Radiology Physics: A Handbook for Teachers and Students* (Vienna: International Atomic Energy Agency)

[4] Balter S 2001 *Interventional Fluoroscopy: Physics, Technology and Safety* (New York: Wiley-Liss)

[5] Rehani M M *et al* 2010 Radiological protection in fluoroscopically guided procedures performed outside the imaging department *Annals of the ICRP* 40, publication 117

[6] Sanchez R, Vano E, Ubeda C, Fernandez J M, Balter S and Hoornaert B 2012 Influence of image metrics when assessing image quality from a test object in cardiac x-ray systems: part II *J. Digit. Imaging Off. J. Soc. Comput. Appl. Radiol.* **25** 537–41

[7] Hart D, Hillier M C and Shrimpton P C 2012 *Doses to Patients from Radiographic and Fluoroscopic X-ray Imaging Procedures in the UK—2010 Review* (Chilton: Health Protection Agency)

[8] Boone J *et al* 1993 A survey of fluoroscopic exposure rates: AAPM Task Group No. 11 report *Med. Phys.* **20** 789–94

[9] International Atomic Energy Agency 2007 Dosimetry in diagnostic radiology: an international code of practice *IAEA Technical Report* No. 457 Vienna, Austria

[10] Rauch P *et al* 2012 Functionality and operation of fluoroscopic automatic brightness control/automatic dose rate control logic in modern cardiovascular and interventional angiography systems: a report of Task Group 125 Radiography/Fluoroscopy Subcommittee, Imaging Physics Committee, Science Council *Med. Phys.* **39** 2826–8

[11] Dehairs M, Bosmans H, Desmet W and Marshall N W 2017 Evaluation of automatic dose rate control for flat panel imaging using a spatial frequency domain figure of merit *Phys. Med. Biol.* **62** 6610–30

[12] Gislason A J, Davies A G and Cowen A R 2010 Dose optimization in pediatric cardiac x-ray imaging *Med. Phys.* **37** 5258

[13] Gislason-Lee A J, McMillan C, Cowen A R and Davies A G 2013 Dose optimization in cardiac x-ray imaging *Med. Phys.* **40** 091911

[14] Gislason-Lee A, Hoornaert B, Cowen A R and Davies A G 2013 Understanding automated dose control in dynamic x-ray imaging systems *European Congress on Radiology (Vienna, Austria, 28 March–1 April 2013)* pp 1–26 https://epos.myesr.org/poster/esr/ecr2013/C-2183/background

[15] Department of Health and Human Services Food and Drug Administration 2005 Electronic products; performance standard for diagnostic x-ray systems and their major components. Final rule *Fed. Regist.* **70** 33997–4042

[16] International Electrotechnical Commission 2010 Medical electrical equipment–part 2-43: Particular requirements for basic safety and essential performance of x-ray equipment for interventional procedures *IEC Standards* IEC 60601-2-43

[17] IPEM 2002 *Medical and Dental Guidance Notes: A Good Practice Guide on all Aspects of Ionising Radiation Protection in the Clinical Environment* (York: IPEM)

[18] IPEM 2019 *Medical and Dental Guidance Notes: A Good Practice Guide on all Aspects of Ionising Radiation Protection in the Clinical Environment* 2nd edn (York: IPEM)

[19] Stewart F A *et al* 2012 ICRP statement on tissue reactions and early and late effects of radiation in normal tissues and organs—threshold doses for tissue reactions in a radiation protection context *Annals of the ICRP* 41, publication 118 pp 1–322

[20] Balter S 2006 Methods for measuring fluoroscopic skin dose *Pediatr. Radiol.* **36** 136–40

[21] Shrimpton P, Wall B, Jones D and Fisher E 1984 The measurement of energy imparted to patients during diagnostic x-ray examinations using the diamentor exposure-area product meter *Phys. Med. Biol.* **29** 1199

[22] British Standard Institution 2010 Medical electrical equipment: particular requirements for the basic safety and essential performance of x-ray equipment for radiography and radioscopy *BSI Standard* BS EN 60601-2-54:2009+A2:2019

[23] Jones A K, Ensor J E and Pasciak A S 2014 How accurately can the peak skin dose in fluoroscopy be determined using indirect dose metrics? *Med. Phys.* **41** 4–11

[24] Neofotistou V *et al* 2003 Preliminary reference levels in interventional cardiology *Eur. Radiol.* **13** 2259–63

[25] Johnson P B, Borrego D, Balter S, Johnson K and Siragusa D 2011 Skin dose mapping for fluoroscopically guided interventions *Med. Phys.* **38** 5490–9

[26] Bordier C, Klausz R and Desponds L 2014 Patient dose map indications on interventional x-ray systems and validation with gafchromic XR-RV3 film *Radiat. Prot. Dosimetry* **163** 306–18

[27] G E Healthcare 2014 Limiting radiation dose in image-guided coronary interventions

[28] Rana V, Rudin S and Bednar D R 2015 A real-time skin dose tracking system for biplane neuro-interventional procedures *Proc. SPIE* **9312** 941230

[29] Orth R, Wallace M and Kuo M 2008 C-arm cone-beam CT: general principles and technical considerations for use in interventional radiology *J. Vasc. Interv. Radiol.* **19** 814–21

[30] Health and Safety Executive 1999 *Guidance Note PM77: Equipment Used in Connection with Medical Exposure* 3rd edn (Sudbury: Health and Safety Executive)

Chapter 3

Radiation protection and tube output tests

3.1 Introduction

Ideally, performance testing should be done in isolation of the other system components. However, this is usually impossible with dynamic systems because the ADRC feedback mechanism is usually hardwired into the system and cannot be decoupled. This is the case even when it is possible to choose the tube potential for the system as the feedback mechanism may still be in partial operation. Testing equipment in these modes can lead to errors as different manufacturers incorporate automatic changes to filters and pulse lengths (or even focus changes) to improve image quality, and the user is rarely aware of these changes. It is clearly easier to test these parameters in an engineering or physics mode (such as the NEMA User QC Mode, see section 2.3.4) if this is available, although extreme care should be taken if operating the system without the normal tube protection systems in place (it is highly unlikely a manufacturer would allow for this to be possible).

Following on from a very brief explanation of the main tests that should be carried out, the rest of the chapter will deal with the differences that must be incorporated into testing the tube and generator on dynamic x-ray equipment. Detailed information about the general testing of tubes and generators can be obtained elsewhere [1].

3.2 Measurements

3.2.1 Half value layer (HVL)

Measurement of the half value layer (HVL) can be difficult in dynamic imaging systems, particularly so if extra filtration is added automatically by the ADRC. The first aim of this test is to ensure the filtration will always exceed the 2.5 mm Al minimum. The anatomical programme with the minimum added spectral filtration available should therefore be chosen for testing. Most modern solid state dosimeters will report the HVL. Reliance on these reported values is the quickest

doi:10.1088/978-0-7503-3819-6ch3

acceptable method to use, provided their accuracy has been validated. HVL can also be measured using the traditional method as described here. This is encouraged even if the dosimeter-reported HVL is within measurement tolerance. Converting from HVL to filtration can be done using the data in IPSM report 64 [2]. Some prefer to test annually, however, the below frequency recommendation is in line with EBQA recommendations [7].

Aims: To ensure that the minimum filtration thickness is greater than 2.5 mm [3, 4] and to ensure that the beam filtration remains constant throughout the working lifespan of the tube.

Frequency: Commissioning only or when filtration material has or could have been altered, i.e. collimator replacement, change in ADRC programming, etc.

Reference value: Minimum 2.5 mm Al filtration.

Remedial level: None.

Suspension level: <2.5 mm Al filtration.

Method: The recommended set-up shown in figure 3.1 can be used to ensure that the ADRC is operating as close as possible to the chosen tube potential and the ADRC remains stable. This is most easily accomplished in the AP projection, adding sheets of aluminium to the II or FP detector at position A until the desired tube voltage is reached; 70 kVp is typically used. It is recommended that the x-ray beam is collimated inside the aluminium squares. In future, using the NEMA UQCM mode [5] the kVp will be able to be set to a specific value rather than what the attenuating thickness drives the ADRC up to.

It is advisable to incorporate the measurement device, preferably a transparent detector or ion chamber (⊕ in figure 3.1) far enough away from A or B to minimise backscatter, and before the aluminium sheets are placed, to stop the ADRC reacting to the presence of the chamber. Once the tube voltage is obtained, moving individual sheets from B to A changes the filtration with respect to the dosimeter, yet the total filtration (beam attenuation measured by the ADRC) remains constant. A plot of air

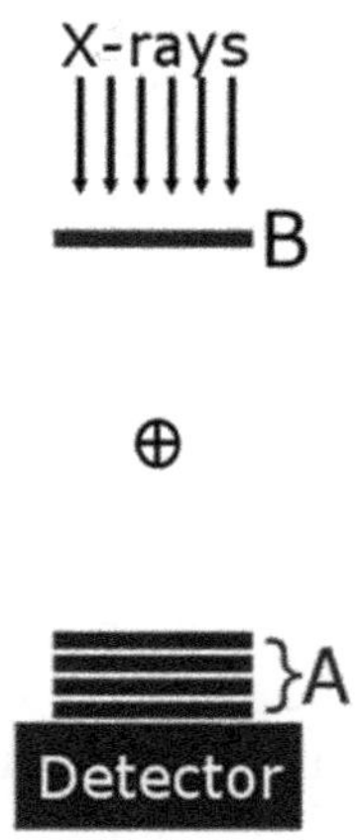

Figure 3.1. Geometric set-up for tube output tests.

KERMA against thickness of aluminium allows the HVL to be calculated. The availability of the NEMA UQCM mode will make this measurement easier and more convenient, probably with increased accuracy [5].

3.2.2 Tube voltage accuracy

Aim: To assess the accuracy of the tube voltage set by the system.

Frequency: 12 monthly.

Remedial level: ±5 % or ±5 kVp, whichever is greater [6].

Suspension level: ±10 % or ±10 kVp, whichever is greater [6].

Method: One of the largest difficulties in measuring tube voltage in a dynamic imaging system is ensuring that the x-ray tube output is sufficient to trigger the measuring instrument. The placement of tube voltage meters close to the x-ray output port to increase the x-ray output to the trigger level will cause an adjustment by the ADRC. Clearly, there is a balance between ensuring sufficient output and the tube voltage selected by the ADRC. From experience, this appears to be easiest by placing the x-ray tube–detector direction laterally and resting the tube voltage meter on a non-attenuating object in the beam. In this way it is simple to adjust the tube voltage by moving the tube voltage meter closer or further away from the tube output port. Additional copper can be placed on the detector face to extend the tube voltage range. It is still important to ensure that measuring device (meter) has the correct orientation with respect to the anode-heel effect on the system. It is important to chose a programme that does not employ additional beam filtration; the beam quality must be within the calibrated range of the kV meter.

A further complication is that some dosimeters will reset before the ADRC has stabilised. However, most modern dosimeters now have methods available to circumvent this issue, either by adding a delay before the measurement starts or by adding a continuous measurement function, and allow the waveform to be plotted.

These waveforms are very useful as they provide an understanding of what the x-ray system is doing. For example, some systems minimise stabilisation time by using the maximum frame rate and then changing to the reported frame rate when stable.

3.2.3 Focal spot

This test was traditionally completed to test the manufacturer-quoted focal spot size is accurate, however, on modern systems the focal spot size is quoted as nominal. Few UK physicists complete this test routinely today [7]. It may be useful as part of an investigation should a problem (for example, a drop in spatial resolution) potentially stem from a change in focal spot. Some may perform it at commissioning to assure a clear understanding of focal spot size in the case of future problems as suggested above. This test is not required for routine follow-up testing.

Test methodology for this assessment can be found in IPEM report 32, part 1 [1]. Focal spot measurements can normally be made using a 1 degree star/spoke test object placed on the tube exit port or patient table and the star imaged and read directly from the monitors, although care should be taken to ensure the acquisition image matrix is of sufficient resolution to give an accurate result. Use of an acquisition (single shot or image sequence) programme rather than fluorostore should ensure this, keeping in mind the effects of unavoidable image processing (which should be less of an issue after NEMA UCQM).

Most systems will automatically choose the focal spot depending on the imaging requirement or clinical programme selected and may not report this to the user. However, as a rule, anatomical programmes designed for patients with a greater habitus will often use the large focus to improve heat dissipation, while fluoroscopy commonly uses fine focus to maintain best possible resolution. On some systems this choice can be set, allowing measurement of all foci at similar radiographic factors. Be aware that on some systems not all tube foci may be enabled. Again, the NEMA user QC mode will make this test easier to perform.

3.2.4 KERMA area product (KAP) and interventional reference point (IRP) air KERMA

The accuracy of the KAP readings provided by the imaging system is important since KAP readings may be used to assess individual patient doses, population doses, or for optimisation purposes. In order to calculate KAP independently of the imaging system, the air KERMA must be measured as well as the x-ray field area in the same plane (the same distance from the focal spot of the x-ray tube). The air KERMA is then multiplied by the area to provide a KAP value which can be compared to that indicated by the system. Note that the air KERMA can be measured using an ion chamber (placed away from sources of scatter) or using a solid state dosimeter (usually placed in the same plane as the field size measurement). The ADRC will be affected by the dosimeter but this will have no effect on the measurement as long as its presence does not shift the kVp to a point higher than the kVp to be tested.

If it is anticipated that the patient image sequences will typically be captured with the x-ray tube below the table, then air KERMA measurements should be made through the table (e.g. an interventional system) using a table transmission factor to correct for the attenuation of the table. If, however, it is expected that the system will typically be used with the tube above the patient and table, or in a lateral position, then dose measurements should be made without the table between x-ray tube and dosimeter. The patient mattress, which sits on the table, should never be included in any measurements. The manufacturer's calibration method should be confirmed at commissioning; failure to follow the manufacturer's calibration protocol has been shown to cause higher failure rates [7].

Aim: To assess the accuracy of the indicated KAP readings.

Frequency: 12 monthly.

Remedial level: Manufacturer recommended tolerance (although some might see these as inappropriate, this is the legally binding tolerance).

Method:

1. An ion chamber (positioned away from scatter with the result corrected for the distance from the tube that the field size was measured) or a solid state

chamber (which can be placed on FPD/II and will affect the ADRC) should be positioned at the centre of the x-ray field free from the effects of scatter.
2. Some attenuating material (e.g. copper) should be positioned on the detector to increase the radiographic factors.
3. The focus to dosimeter and SID distances should be measured and recorded.
4. The accumulated KAP and air KERMA values indicated by the system should be recorded.
5. In order to quickly accumulate a statistically significant measured air KERMA and indicated air KERMA and KAP, it is recommended that a relatively high dose and pulse rate mode is selected.
6. Expose for a long enough period to allow a significant change in the indicated KAP and air KERMA values.
7. Record the accumulated dose from the dosimeter, as well as the indicated KAP and air KERMA values (subtracting the starting values as appropriate).
8. The area of the irradiated field should be measured at the same distance from the focal spot as the air KERMA measurement was made in, if practically feasible; this can be done with a computed radiography (CR) cassette of appropriate size. Otherwise it can be measured at a different distance and corrected for using the inverse square law.
9. The measured KAP is calculated by multiplying the measured field area by the measured air KERMA (either measured or corrected to the same plane) and then compared to the indicated values.
10. The measured air KERMA should be distance corrected to the IRP before being compared to the indicated air KERMA.

3.2.5 Radiation to image field size (area)

Aim: To assess the degree of overlap of the radiation field to the image area.

Frequency: 12 monthly.

Remedial level: Ratio of radiation field area to captured image field area > 1.15.

Suspension level: Radiation field outside of detector housing.

Method:

1. Position a CR cassette (or Gafchromic film or similar) in front of the detector.
2. Measure the focus to CR cassette distance as well as the SID.
3. Place markers on the CR plate to indicate the limit of the detector housing.
4. Expose the CR cassette to fluoroscopy for approximate 1 s on each FOV, ensuring in each case that the collimators are open to their full allowable extent.
5. Read the CR image and use software distance measuring tools to measure dimensions, before calculating the area of each x-ray field.
6. Compare the measured areas to the image areas calculated from measurements taken using Leeds test object M1. If the image area and irradiated

area are measured in different planes, ensure that appropriate distance corrections are made.

3.2.6 Image field size

Aim: Compare the displayed field of view versus nominal diameter.

Frequency: 12 monthly for IITV, acceptance test for FP detectors.

Remedial level: Measured FOV within ±15% of nominal FOV [7].

Method:

1. Set largest FOV, clinical default fluoroscopy mode.
2. Centre the Leeds M1 test object at image detector input plane and measure focus–M_1 distance.
3. Perform fluoroscopy briefly to obtain the LIH of the TO.
4. Count the number of squares seen in the x- and y-directions to give measured field size in cm.
5. Correct for any difference in magnification between focus (M_1) distance and focus–image detector input distance:

   $FOV_{true} = FOV_{meas}$(focus to x-ray converter dist.)÷(focus to M_1 TO dist.).
6. Compare to nominal field size.
7. Repeat for all FOVs.
8. For fields larger than M_1, measure the diameter of M_1 on the display in cm for the x- and y-directions. Calculate the magnification (M_1= 25 cm). Measure the diameter of the display (or TV blanking circle) and divide the display diameter by the magnification to obtain the observed field size.
9. For IITV systems, expect FOV_{true} to be within 20% (x%) of the nominal FOV; for FP-based systems, expect FOV_{true} to be within 10% (y%) of the nominal FOV. See the national survey data for [8].

3.3 Dosimetry tests

3.4 Dosimeter selection

There are three types of device that could be chosen to measure DAKR and ESAKR:

- Ionisation chambers coupled to electrometers.
- Solid state dosimeter with lead backing.
- Transparent solid state dosimeter (without lead backing).

A thorough discussion of the first two options is provided by Martin *et al* [9]. The lead backing will largely eliminate backscatter reaching the solid state detector. Consequently a correction factor may need to be applied if trying to compare to measurements made with an ionisation chamber system. It is important to consider this effect when making comparisons, for example to published reference data, to limits or guidance, or to service engineer measurements if different types of dose measurement devices have been used.

If a solid state dosimeter with lead backing is to be used, then care must be taken over positioning. If located within the ADRC's sensitive area then a reduction of the sampled signal may occur, which may cause a change in x-ray factors and DAKR. This may be the case to a lesser extent with some ionisation chambers as well. The ADRC sensing region can cover the entire image on many modern systems so this it is difficult to avoid this. However, the influence of the meter on ADRC factors may be small. It is important to take care to ensure that the set-up is reproducible to allow meaningful comparison to the baseline.

Lead (or similar material) backed dosimeters can still be used but care is needed, in particular on smaller FOVs where it has a larger influence. In order to assess the effect of a lead backed dosimeter, the radiographic factors should be compared with and without the dosimeter in the field. If a large difference is seen then this should be noted. One option could be to select a different ADRC sensing region, which is not always possible.

Transparent solid state dosimeters are a more recent addition to the market and may obviate some of the problems caused by the lead backing, however, at the time of writing there was limited experience with their use. It is known that some such systems attempt to correct for backscatter and it is important to understand how such a measurement device is working before use.

Where a lead backed dosimeter is used, a backscatter factor is required to correct to the true ESDR. This value could be determined locally based on phantom material and local testing methodology. Backscatter correction values will typically be in the range of 1.2–1.5, but are dependent on field size, beam quality, filtration, and scattering medium and thickness. A value of 1.4 is appropriate for 80 kVp, filtered with 4.0 mm Al in a 20 cm wide x-ray field [10]. For a more complete examination of backscatter factors see IPSM report 53 'Patient Dosimetry Techniques in Diagnostic Radiology' [11]. In a department where different types of dosimeters are used, correction between different dosimeters can be problematic and therefore it is easier to use a single detector type (for example ion chambers only) in dynamic imaging QA. If the department requires different dosimeters to be used on the same dynamic imaging system, some work should be undertaken to correct for the different environments in which the DAKR is measured.

3.5 Detector air KERMA rate (DAKR)

Detector (input) air KERMA rate DAKR has in the past been measured [12] with a 1 mm thick copper sheet at the tube exit port and an ionisation chamber at the surface of the image detector (with the grid removed where possible). On modern systems under ADRC operation, the use of a 1 mm thick copper attenuator may lead to a low tube voltage (commonly less than 60 kVp), which can influence the measured DAKR [13]. Furthermore, if the Leeds test objects are used for detector image quality evaluation, then a low tube voltage may lie outside the range for which contrast data is available. Consequently it is recommended that a thickness of 2 mm copper is chosen as a starting point.

If the use of 2 mm copper results in the ADRC selecting a tube voltage outside the range of 65–80 kVp, then it is recommended that the copper thickness is varied to achieve tube voltages in this range. Threshold contrast tables are provided for 1.0, 1.5, and 2.0 mm copper by Leeds test objects. The thickness of copper chosen will have only a small effect on the measured dose rates, caused by the small variation in detector sensitivity as a function of tube voltage within the range of interest [14, 15]. It is, however, advisable that the chosen thickness of copper is maintained over successive years of testing.

Furthermore, it is important to ensure that all copper sheets in the QC kit have equal thickness. The usual tolerance on copper plate is ±0.1 mm without excessive cost. This will have little effect on the DAKR measurement, but it will change the tube voltage and current that the ADRC sets, which may influence conclusions drawn when comparing to previous values. This tolerance also assumes that the same copper sheet (or sheets from the same batch known to be consistent) is used for the lifetime of the system to ensure consistency.

3.5.1 Method for measuring DAKR

Aim: To assess the DAKR so that it can be compared to expected levels at commissioning and subsequently compared to baseline. DAKR is an important parameter when viewing image quality results and considering optimisation strategies.

Frequency: 12 monthly.

Method:

1. Set the SID to a predefined value. The exact distance is not of key importance, but keeping the distance constant over consecutive tests is. This allows a meaningful comparison of settings chosen by the ADRC between sets of consecutive measurements. Consideration should be given to whether measurements should be done with the table in the field or otherwise. Again, it is not a crucial decision, but consistency aids meaningful comparisons.
2. The copper thickness should be chosen at commissioning such that the system chooses a tube voltage between 65 and 80 kVp, and positioned at the tube exit port. Ideally, the same copper sheet should be used to mitigate changes in thickness due to manufacturing tolerances.
3. The aim of this test is to estimate the DAKR at the input plane of image detector, hence the grid should be removed where possible. Measuring with the grid out allows a more meaningful comparison to be made between the detector performance between systems and with published data. If this is not possible, then efforts should be made to determine a grid attenuation correction factor. It may be possible to measure the grid factor at commissioning with the assistance of an engineer, and then be applied to the results in subsequent years. Alternatively the manufacturer may be able to supply this factor. Typical primary beam grid attenuation factors for dynamic x-ray systems are in the range 1.4–1.7. In the absence of any information about the

primary beam grid attenuation factor, it is recommended that a factor of 1.5 is used as a default.

4. The dosimeter should be positioned on the surface of the detector housing. If using an ion chamber, or transparent solid state detector, then the dosimeter can be positioned in the centre of the field. See the comments in section 4.3.2 on positioning of the dosimeter with respect to the ADRC sensing region. It is good practice to adopt a consistent methodology regarding the position of the dosimeter as this can have some influence on the result.
5. The clinical programme and fluoroscopy mode should be noted.
6. The dosimeter should be set in a mode that will report dose rate. After the fluoroscopy exposure is initiated, a few seconds should be allowed for the radiographic factors and measured dose rate to stabilise, before a dose rate and factors (kV, mA, pulse width, added filtration) can be recorded. If the chosen fluoroscopy mode has a frame rate below 7.5 fps, it may be difficult to achieve a stable, reliable dose rate reading, depending on the integration time of the dosimeter. If this is the case then it may be preferable to record accumulated dose over a short period (e.g. 10 s) to estimate dose rate (if the dosimeter has such a function).
7. DAKR can be measured for acquisition sequences in exactly the same manner as for the fluoroscopy sequence. On rare occasions it may be that a different copper thickness is necessary to achieve tube voltages in the desired range in acquisition from that necessary in fluoroscopy.
8. For each DAKR measurement it is recommended that where possible the following parameters are recorded: clinical mode (programme), dose rate mode, frame rate, FOV, tube voltage, mA, pulse length (ms), filtration added by the system, grid status (in or out), and DAKR.

3.5.2 Range of DAKR tests at commissioning

3.5.2.1 DAKR variation with field size

A commonly used (in the clinical setting of the x-ray system being tested) anatomical programme should be selected. Using the default fluoroscopy setting the DAKR should be measured in each field size in turn and repeated in acquisition. Traditionally, image intensifiers were set up such that when magnification settings varied, DAKR would increase inversely proportionally with the area of the chosen field size. This was necessary in order to maintain constant light photon flux reaching the intensifier output phosphor. On modern II systems, this relationship may still hold true, but there is no longer an absolute requirement to maintain light photon flux reaching the output phosphor as a constant. Consequently, some systems may behave differently. FP systems will almost certainly not behave in this way, with many current FP-based systems modulating DAKR as 1/FOV, with the aim of maintaining perceived noise within some acceptable level. Note that the pre-programmed variation of DAKR can often be found in the system (service) settings or system documentation.

3.5.2.2 Programmes and modes

Within one clinical programme, systems will have several fluoroscopy modes, with nomenclatures varying between manufacturers: Fluoro 1, Fluoro 2, and Fluoro 3, or low dose, normal, and high quality. Additionally, there may also be several different acquisition modes associated with the anatomical programme. DAKR should be measured in all these modes for a single FOV. The chosen FOV should ideally be that commonly used clinically (i.e. choose ~20 cm when assessing cardiac systems). This should be repeated for the commonly used anatomical programmes.

3.5.2.3 Frame rates

On some systems frame rates may only be adjustable by varying anatomical programmes or dose rate modes. If it is possible to independently adjust frame rates, then within the chosen anatomical programme, for the field size chosen, DAKR should be measured for a range of frame rates, both in fluoroscopy and acquisition—do this at the commissioning stage. It is not necessarily expected or appropriate for DAKR to be proportional to frame rate in either fluoroscopy or acquisition modes.

At low frame rates (of the order of 5 fps or lower), if the air KERMA per frame is constant then halving of the frame rate will also half the DAKR. However, the perceived image quality (contrast resolution) for both frame rates will be approximately constant. This is because the human visual system is unable to perform frame averaging over a time range of more than 200 ms, i.e. individual frames will be assessed by the brain as individual images.

Other systems will be set up to increase the dose per frame when the frame rate is lowered to maintain perceived image quality. Aufrichtig *et al* [16] reported that in order to maintain image quality when decreasing the frame rate from 30 fps to 15 fps, the air KERMA per frame had to be increased by a factor of 1.6. Similarly, at 10 fps and 7.5 fps dose per frame increase factors of 1.78 and 1.87 were required to maintain comparable image quality at 30 fps. It is important to note that the use of pulsed imaging modes is absolutely recommended and there is still a net reduction in 'dose' when using pulsed imaging, it is just that this reduction is not as large as might be expected from the (naïve) expectation that dose/frame is kept constant as pulse rate is adjusted. It should be noted that this analysis holds true for static objects only. For moving objects, higher frame rates will of course allow for clearer visualisation of movement.

3.5.3 Expected dose rates and their intended clinical use

Consideration of the initial dose rate set-up should involve a multidisciplinary team including medical physics expert [17], radiographers, the manufacturer applications specialist, and the clinicians/radiographers involved in image interpretation and acquisition. It is not possible or meaningful to define a single set of expected dose rates for all fluoroscopy and image acquisition because it is entirely dependent on the clinical task. Note that some current systems and future ADRC systems may not have target DAKR levels; DAKR is just another parameter (along with kV, mA, ms, focus size, spectral filtration) that is modulated such that the target image quality level is achieved [18]. See table 3.1 for commissioning test tolerances

One resource that is useful is to compare doses measured in existing rooms that perform similar procedures (including the room being replaced). For similar anatomical programmes or modes, DAKR levels that are notably higher or lower should be questioned, investigated, and justified. In considering the optimisation of low dose fluoroscopy settings, it is important to be aware of the difference in noise properties between FP detectors and image intensifiers.

A well set-up II should approximately maintain its DQE over the full range of clinically relevant doses. In the past FP-based systems could suffer from a reduction in DQE at very low doses per frame due to additive electronic noise. In the

Table 3.1. Commissioning test tolerances. Values should be compared to manufacturer specification. In this context manufacturer specification should be taken to mean the dose levels programmed into the system with the agreement of the MPE in conjunction with clinical colleagues. It is not the manufacturer's responsibility to define dose levels that the system must operate at.

Test	Remedial level	Suspension level
DAKR variation with magnification	All measured dose rates should be within 25% of the manufacturer's specification, taking into account methodological differences. The ratio of DAKR between two field sizes different from the manufacturer's specification, or expected relationship—at the MPE's discretion.	All measured dose rates should be within 50% of the manufacturer's specification taking into account methodological differences—at the MPE's discretion.
DAKR variation with dose rate modes	All dose rate modes should be different to each other with dose rate logically increasing from low dose mode to high (as opposed to vice versa). All measured dose rates should be within 25% of the manufacturer's specification, taking into account methodological differences.	All measured dose rates should be within 50% of the manufacturer's specification taking into account methodological differences—at the MPE's discretion.
DAKR variation with frame modes	All measured dose rates should be within 25% of the manufacturer's specification, taking into account methodological differences.	All measured dose rates should be within 50% of the manufacturer's specification, taking into account methodological differences.
DAKR variation with clinical modes	All measured dose rates should be within 25% of the manufacturer's specification, taking into account methodological differences.	All measured dose rates should be within 50% of the manufacturer's specification, taking into account methodological differences.

fluoroscopy dose range some loss in DQE with decreasing dose is expected, leading to a disproportionate loss of image quality at very low DAKR [19]. Particular care should be taken if reducing the dose per frame to the order of 10 nGy.

3.5.4 Quality control (QC) testing

Following commissioning tests, periodic QC tests should be performed, comparing results to baseline measurements. The following tests are recommended.

3.5.4.1 Field of view

For the anatomical programme chosen at commissioning, DAKR should be measured for a range of FOVs. Some modern FP systems can have up to eight field sizes and there is little value in testing them all—a representative range of field sizes is sufficient.

3.5.4.2 Dose rate modes

The full range of dose rate modes should be tested for one FOV in at least one commonly used clinical mode. The clinical mode(s) chosen should be matched to that tested at commissioning for comparison. QC test tolerances are summarised in table 3.2.

3.5.4.3 Frame rates

Within a single clinical mode, dose rate mode and field size (all matched to that chosen at commissioning), DAKR should be measured every few years for a range of frame rates (if it is possible to independently vary frame rate). This can be done for fluoroscopy and acquisition modes. Provided there were no major programming changes made by a manufacturer engineer or applications specialist since commissioning (these can be delivered from offsite), there should be no need for these follow-up measurements.

3.5.4.4 Anatomical programmes

In the default anatomical programme and chosen FOV, fluoroscopy DAKR should be measured for a range of common programmes. The range tested will depend on the system and available time, but is expected to be a much smaller range than tested at commissioning and should be limited to modes in common clinical use. Similarly acquisition DAKR should be measured in a range of clinical modes.

Table 3.2. QC test tolerances.

Test	Remedial level	Suspension level
DAKR variation with FOV	Baseline ± 25%	Baseline ± 50%
DAKR variation with dose rate modes	Baseline ± 25%	Baseline ± 50%
DAKR variation with clinical modes	Baseline ± 25%	Baseline ± 50%

3.6 Patient entrance surface air KERMA rate (ESAKR)

Modern interventional systems (those produced since 2010) will conform to the requirements of the current IEC standard for safety and performance of interventional x-ray equipment which requires the live display of patient dose rate at the IRP and cumulative air KERMA delivered to this point over the course of a procedure (section 2.2.5). Although most manufacturers will support both the IEC and the FDA IRPs, equipment installed in the UK should comply with the IEC standard.

Measurements of patient ESAKR are conventionally made at the surface of a phantom in the position normally occupied by the patient such that backscatter can also be included in the measurement made. However, if measurements are made solely for comparison with reported doses (at the IRP) then scatter is not required as systems will report air KERMA at this position. For these measurements, any low backscatter attenuator may be used at the image detector, e.g. a copper sheet.

3.6.1 Phantom materials

The choice of phantom material will largely be dictated by what is locally available to the physicist. If a patient equivalent phantom is to be used, to include backscatter, the material should be close to tissue equivalence to accurately simulate backscatter towards the measurement chamber, so tissue equivalent material (TEM), water, and PMMA are acceptable. PMMA is between 6% and 11% more attenuating than water to a 70 kVp x-ray beam depending on beam filtration (see appendix A.3). An acceptable correction for fluoroscopy systems is 90 mm PMMA to 100 mm water.

The phantom should ideally be of sufficient size to cover the entire captured image area in the largest FOV to avoid collimating if possible or at least sufficient to cover the ADRC sensing area. For most systems 25 cm × 25 cm blocks will be sufficient. Thicknesses of 20, 30, and 40 cm water-equivalent material is recommended at commissioning, ideally in 2.5, 5, or 10 cm thick sections that can be used for the testing of other thickness. For paediatric systems, 5 or 10 cm thicknesses should be tested in addition to greater thicknesses. If testing skin dose rates on mini C-arms (which are used for imaging thin body sections such as hands and fingers) 5 cm is a common choice of attenuator thickness.

3.6.2 Method for measuring ESAKR

1. Position a scatter phantom of 20 cm water-equivalent thickness in the x-ray beam path with the beam incident perpendicular to the phantom surface. Ideally the positioning should also simulate some characteristics of the patient position clinically, e.g. the beam should pass through the table before the phantom if that would be the typical clinical set-up. The phantom will need to be raised above the table to allow for positioning of the dosimeter between the phantom and the table, i.e. at the entrance surface of the phantom. For mobile fluoroscopy systems where the system is tested without a table present, it may be easier to position the system laterally with the phantom placed on

a trolley or stand. Heavy phantoms should not be placed directly on the image detector as this can distort the C-arm.

2. Set the SID to a predefined value consistent with previous testing on the system. Keeping the distance constant over consecutive years of testing is essential to maintaining an accurate record of system performance through time and allows the reported settings chosen by the ADRC to be meaningfully compared between sets of consecutive measurements. When initially choosing an SID, a clinically representative value is preferred [20]. A gap of 10–15 cm between the phantom and the front face of the image detector housing will be consistent with clinical practice. Placement of the phantom entrance at the IRP will also allow the dose at the interventional reference point to be measured directly. This would mean that all phantom thicknesses below 30 cm would be less than that IRP and those larger would be higher than the IRP. The IRP is not necessarily at 65 cm from the x-ray source; it depends where the isocentre is and therefore is not fixed.
3. If the grid has been removed for the previous test, ensure the grid is in place now (i.e. as used clinically).
4. The dosimeter should be positioned on the phantom surface facing towards the x-ray beam. If using an ion chamber, or transparent solid state detector, then the dosimeter can be positioned in the centre of the field. If using a lead backed solid state detector, then care is required to avoid placing it over part of the sensing area of the ADRC. The dosimeter should be set in a mode that will report dose rate. After the fluoroscopy exposure is initiated, a few seconds should be allowed for the radiographic factors and measured dose rate to stabilise, before a dose rate, factors (kV, mA, frame width, spectral filtration), and reported dose rate can be recorded. If the chosen fluoroscopy mode has a low frame rate (below ~5 fps), it may be difficult to achieve a stable and reliable live dose rate reading, depending on the integration time of the dosimeter. If this is the case, then it may be preferable to record accumulated dose over a short period (e.g. 10 s) to estimate dose rate (if the dosimeter has such a function).
5. ESAKR can be measured for acquisition sequences in exactly the same manner as for the fluoroscopy sequence, but dose per frame should be recorded (figure 3.2).

3.6.3 Range of ESAKR tests at commissioning

The same range of dose rate modes, field sizes, and frame rates should be assessed for ESAKR as for DAKR, with priority given to combinations likely to be in common use and to result in higher patient doses. At the MPE's discretion it may not be necessary to test this full range of parameters for both DAKR and ESAKR. In addition, the performance of the system when imaging should include a range of phantom thicknesses. This will depend on the clinical use of the system, but for most interventional and cardiology systems it would not be unreasonable to include water-equivalent phantom thicknesses up to 40 cm.

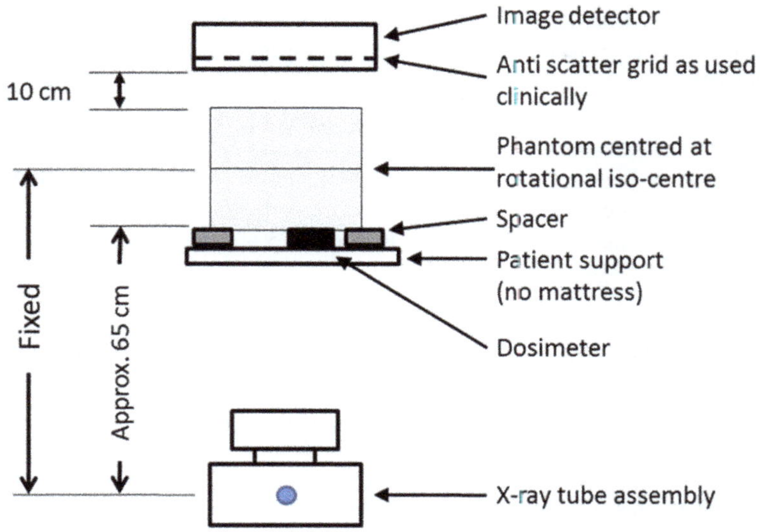

Figure 3.2. Example of a set-up for ESAKR measurement. Measurement is made with a dosimeter on the surface of a phantom facing the x-ray tube.

This is not only to reflect potential patient size in the PA direction, but also the oblique views commonly used in these clinical areas. It is also useful to measure the maximum ESAKR that can be delivered by the system in both fluoroscopy and acquisition modes. This should be assessed by placing a lead attenuator, such as a double thickness of lead apron, behind the phantom but before the image detector such that backscatter is still included in the measurement (if this is desired).

Some physicists may be interested in the effect of collimation on ESAKR [7], measuring it with a range of collimations at commissioning to understand how the ADRC responds to collimation for a given x-ray system. It is for the MPE to decide whether this test is necessary to help identify how the ADRC responds to collimation.

3.6.4 Comparison to system-reported air KERMA rates

Aim: To allow a comparison of the system-reported air KERMA rates to those measured and determine the position of the patient entrance reference point (IEC interventional reference point) for the system to be measured as a distance from the x-ray source. Test tolerances are summarised in table 3.3.

The IEC interventional reference point (see figure 2.7) is defined at 15 cm to tube side of isocentre for C-arm models. For undercouch systems the reference level is defined as 1 cm above the patient support, or 30 cm above the patient support for overcouch units (IEC 60601-2-43 edn 2). The FDA defined an alternative reference point at 30 cm from the detector face. Doses measured using the method described in section 4.3.2 may be compared directly with those reported by the system if they were measured in the absence of scatter (or if the scatter component has been estimated and removed) and if a distance correction using the inverse square law has

Table 3.3. Table of test tolerances. Note that these apply to normal largest field size, using a 20 cm water-equivalent phantom, 15 fps frame rate, and largest FOV, so under different experimental conditions results should be interpreted.

Test	Remedial level	Suspension level
ESAKR at the largest FOV	20 mGy min^{-1}	50 mGy min^{-1}
Accuracy of reported dose	25%	35%
All ESAKR measurements	Baseline ±25%	Baseline ±50%

been applied. The IEC tolerance for this value is ±35%, but as substantial error in this calculation is from KAP calibration, systems with a KAP calibration factor close to 1 should achieve a much higher degree of accuracy.

3.6.5 Expected values of ESAKR

The range of skin dose rates observed will vary significantly with patient thickness and clinical application, however, ADRC systems are designed to keep these dose rates below specific set limits, as explained in section 2.2.

The question may be raised whether QC testing of ESAKR should be necessary following commissioning during QA if DAKR measurements are found to be in tolerance, if the programme parameters remain unchanged. Physicists may wish to undertake ESAKR measurements following a change in the system configuration where the DAKR settings have been changed. Some physicists may use ESAKR rather than DAKR as the preferred routine measurement after commissioning. Often a change in one is not reflected on the other in terms of proportionality, therefore it is recommended to use both for routine measurements. The EBQA results suggested that a single result for DAKR or ESAKR was not indicative of the other [8].

3.6.6 Measuring ADRC curves

Aim: To see how the ADRC responds as a function of patient thickness.

Frequency: Commissioning only, and as the need arises as a tool for optimisation, or to investigate changes highlighted by other tests.

Method:

1. Capture a fluoroscopy exposure in the mode chosen with an attenuator in the beam with thickness smaller or equal in size to the thinnest body section likely to be imaged (e.g. 2.5 cm PMMA or 0.5 mm Cu). Ideally this would be PMMA or water phantoms in the patient position. Copper at the tube exit port will enable the same curve to be plotted, but relating the curve to patient sizes will be harder.
2. Record the focus size, tube voltage, tube current, pulse width (if available), and spectral filtration.
3. Add a chosen thickness of attenuating material. Repeat step 2.

4. Add more attenuation to plot additional points on the curve. 2.5 cm steps are recommended if using PMMA or water. Attenuation should continue to be added until the system's maximum factors are reached.
5. Curves similar to those in figures 2.2 and 2.3 should be plotted. This should be repeated for the fluoroscopy and acquisition modes of interest.

It may be possible to plot a limited kV mA^{-1} curve based on the measurements made for the DAKR and ESAKR.

References

[1] Cranley K 1997 Measurement of the performance characteristics of diagnostic x-ray systems used in medicine: x-ray tubes and generators *IPEM Report* 32 (I) 2nd edn, York, UK

[2] Cranley K, Gilmore B and Fogarty G 1991 Data for estimating x-ray tube total filtration *IPSM Report* 64 York, UK

[3] ICRP 1982 Protection against ionizing radiation from external sources used in medicine *Ann. ICRP* **6** IFC

[4] International Electrotechnical Commission 1996 Evaluation and routine testing in medical imaging departments—part 3.3: acceptance tests—imaging performance of x-ray equipment for digital subtraction angiography (DSA) *IEC Report* 61223-3-3:1996 Geneva, Switzerland

[5] NEMA 2018 X-ray equipment for interventional procedures user quality control mode *NEMA Standards Publication* XR 27-2013 (R2018) Rosslyn, VA

[6] Hiles P A, Mackenzie A, Scally A and Wall B 2005 Recommended standards for the routine performance testing of diagnostic x-ray imaging systems *IPEM Report* 91 York, UK

[7] Worrall M *et al* 2019 IPEM topical report: an evidence and risk assessment based analysis of the efficacy of quality assurance tests on fluoroscopy units-part I: dosimetry and safety *Phys. Med. Biol.* **64** 195011

[8] Shaw D *et al* 2020 IPEM topical report: an evidence and risk assessment based analysis of the efficacy of quality assurance tests on fluoroscopy units—part II: image quality *Phys. Med. Biol.* **65** 225037

[9] Martin C J 2007 An evaluation of semiconductor and ionization chamber detectors for diagnostic x-ray dosimetry measurements *Phys. Med. Biol.* **52** 4465–80

[10] Martin C J 1995 Measurement of patient entrance surface dose rates for fluoroscopic x-ray units *Phys. Med. Biol.* **40** 823–34

[11] Wall B, Harrison R and Spiers F 1988 Patient dosimetry techniques in diagnostic radiology *IPSM Report* 53 London, UK

[12] Hiles P A and Starritt H C 1996 Measurement of the performance characteristics of diagnostic x-ray systems used in medicine: x-ray image intensifier television systems *IPEM Report* 32, part 2 York, UK

[13] Boone J *et al* 1993 A survey of fluoroscopic exposure rates: AAPM Task Group No. 11 report *Med. Phys.* **20** 789–94

[14] Reilly A and Sutton D 2001 A computer model of an image intensifier system working under automatic brightness control *Br. J. Radiol.* **74** 938–48

[15] Doyle P and Martin C 2006 Calibrating automatic exposure control devices for digital radiography *Phys. Med. Biol.* **51** 5475–85

[16] Aufrichtig R, Thomas C W, Xue P and Wilson D L 1994 Model for perception of pulsed fluoroscopy image sequences *J. Opt. Soc. Am.* A **11** 3167–76

[17] European Commission 2014 European guidelines on medical physics expert *Radiation Protection Report* No 174 Luxembourg

[18] Dehairs M, Bosmans H, Desmet W and Marshall N W 2017 Evaluation of automatic dose rate control for flat panel imaging using a spatial frequency domain figure of merit *Phys. Med. Biol.* **62** 6610–30

[19] Antonuk L E *et al* Feb. 2000 Strategies to improve the signal and noise performance of active matrix, flat-panel imagers for diagnostic x-ray applications *Med. Phys.* **27** 289–306

[20] Martin C J, Sutton D G, Workman A, Shaw A J and Temperton D Dec. 1998 Protocol for measurement of patient entrance surface dose rates for fluoroscopic x-ray equipment *Br. J. Radiol.* **71** 1283–7

Chapter 4

Technical image quality tests

This section describes some of the methods used to assess the technical image quality of dynamic imaging systems. Some of the most significant contributions in this area have been made by the group at the University of Leeds [1–3]. This has resulted in the Leeds test objects and the associated techniques used to assess image quality being adopted as the de facto standard in the UK. Alternative phantoms and testing approaches have been developed. For example, the Center for Devices and Radiological Health (CDRH), USA, has described a fluoroscopy phantom for use in QC and national surveys [4], while the Deutsches Institute für Normung (DIN) specify standards for x-ray equipment (constancy) testing and phantoms compliant to these standards, and are available from various manufacturers for routine testing. However, given the significant cost implications of new tests objects and the familiarity of physicists with these methods, the Leeds test objects are used where possible in this report. This section begins with a review of the various methods and phantoms used for the performance testing of dynamic imaging systems.

4.1 Factors influencing technical image quality in dynamic imaging

As with other medical x-ray devices, it is useful to consider dynamic imaging systems as a chain of components, each influencing, to a greater or lesser extent, the quality of the images produced by the entire system. Each manufacturer has their own design criteria, with the consequence that there are potentially large differences in performance between systems and components. Some of these parameters are design parameters (for example pixel spacing, TV camera type, x-ray convertor thickness, etc) and cannot be changed, others are settings that can be altered by the applications engineer or operator (target image KERMA rate, FOV, frame rate, etc) and hence are flexible/changeable.

The following gives a flavour of the range of parameters and influencing factors.

doi:10.1088/978-0-7503-3819-6ch4

4.1.1 X-ray tube

X-rays are generated over a finite region and this acts as a source of geometric blurring; the degree of blurring present within the projection images depends on the size of the focus and the geometric magnification. For image runs containing moving anatomy, the duration over which x-rays are produced (the pulse length) is another factor influencing the sharpness of the projection images. The shape of the focus is important: square foci will give isotropic sharpness, while rectangular foci will give images that are sharper in a certain direction. The tube voltage at which the x-ray tube is operated and added spectral filtration affect the primary contrast of the anatomy being captured and are governed by the ADRC control curves.

4.1.2 Scattered radiation and scatter rejection methods

Scattered radiation reduces the contrast of anatomical structures; it also acts as a source of quantum noise, reducing the DQE of the system as a whole [5]. Anti-scatter grids are the standard method used in fluoroscopy systems. Important parameters are the grid total transmission, the grid primary transmission, and signal-to-noise and distortion ratio (SNDR) (or image) improvement factor [6]. The air gap technique is also used, primarily in paediatric imaging.

4.1.3 X-ray image detector (IITV)

The parameters relating to the detector that influence system image quality are many and include input phosphor and photocathode (material composition, physical structure, thickness), pre-sampling MTF of the II components, lag, conversion factor, gain (aperture setting), dynamic range, FOV, veiling glare of the output window, vignetting, fixed pattern noise (input and output phosphors), and TV camera (target composition, MTF, dynamic range, lag, ghosting, gamma, bandwidth, additive electronic noise).

4.1.4 X-ray detector (FPD)

Important parameters again include the x-ray converter (material composition, physical structure, thickness, pre-sampling MTF), detector element spacing, geometric fill factor, gain, detector binning mode, FOV, additive electronic noise, dynamic range, fixed pattern noise, and frame rate (array read-out speed). Image retention (build up lag, decay lag) and ghosting of the x-ray converter and pixel array affects the stochastic and fixed pattern noise present in the image.

4.1.5 Image processing

The scope of image processing used in dynamic imaging systems is enormous and is fundamental to the quality of images produced. Hundreds of parameters and settings are available, for example governing the balance between sharpness and noise (multi-scale filtering, edge enhancement, applied noise reduction including recursive filtering, and motion detection), contrast and brightness, and adaptive dynamic range.

4.1.6 Image display

Influential parameters include the display grayscale calibration (GSDF), minimum and maximum display brightness (contrast ratio), brightness uniformity, temporal response (lag), focus uniformity, pixel size, and viewing angle.

4.1.7 Image viewing conditions

Factors such as ambient illuminance, reflections on the screen, and viewing distance have a direct influence on image quality results acquired using subjective test objects.

4.2 Approaches to image quality assessment in dynamic imaging

The factors listed in section 4.1 give a flavour of the complexity of dynamic imaging systems and the difficulties involved when trying to assess either technical image quality or the final clinical image quality. In fact, the term image quality requires careful definition if we are to be clear what exactly is being quantified and for what purpose. In this document, we consider images of high intrinsic quality to be sharp, with high contrast, and low noise and lag (temporal smearing). However, in medical imaging, images are always produced for some purpose and hence can contain increased noise or lag and still be of sufficient quality to perform the clinical task. This is the notion of task based assessment of image quality [7, 8]—the sharpness, noise (and thus dose), etc of the images produced by the imaging system should be matched to the clinical task.

This ties in with the immense flexibility of the current generation of dynamic imaging systems, where many factors can be changed to result in a wide range of (technical) image quality levels. These systems can be tuned to a particular imaging task, with some required level of sharpness, noise, FOV, and applied lag (which can be adjusted by setting the level of recursive filtering), to obtain sufficient (and no more) quality such that the task can be performed. Hence, one of the tasks of the medical physicist lies in helping to match the different (programmable) levels of technical image quality to the clinical tasks performed on the system. One could therefore argue that technical image quality should be assessed using test objects that simulate the specific task to be performed on the system in question. The problem is that such test objects are limited in terms of scope/task and even if available, would probably have to be evaluated by a clinician (although evaluation by a numerical (or model) observer may be possible in the future). Furthermore, this strays outside the realm of QC and into optimisation; although we consider that these two procedures should be linked.

For the purposes of QC, images of test objects are acquired under controlled conditions in order to assess technical image quality (image sharpness, contrast, lag, noise) of the imaging system and/or components in the imaging chain. At commissioning, results are compared against reference data for typical dynamic imaging systems to give an idea of total system or component performance using these test objects for the fluoroscopy/acquisition programme being assessed. One must be aware of the limitations of commonly used static fluoroscopy test objects when assessing imaging systems set up to image the dynamic content of clinical examinations, in particular the rapidly moving anatomy in cardiac sequences. For routine QC, results acquired using these test objects during a survey visit are compared against baseline data, i.e. data acquired at the commissioning stage or after changes to the protocols/programmes, for example in an optimisation step. This is done in order to isolate problems, changes in performance, drift etc. Test object based evaluation of technical image quality can be broken down into two geometric set-ups, as follows.

4.2.1 Image detector based technical image quality evaluation

In this particular set-up, test objects are placed at the image detector with the intention of minimising the influence of other system factors on the measurement (e.g. x-ray focus size, object motion, x-ray scattered radiation) and isolating detector imaging performance as shown in figure 4.1, where the distances shown can be varied as required to simulate the clinical set-up used.

A similar geometry is adopted when making quantitative detector measurements [9, 10]. This type of test object is often used at a calibrated beam energy, in conjunction with metal (copper and/or aluminium) filtration placed at the x-ray tube so that the influence of tube voltage (energy) is minimised and the contrasts are known with reasonable accuracy.

Advantages of this set-up include the fact that a similar geometry can be used by a physics service for all detectors and that detector performance can be tested against existing standards acquired with the same geometry and tracked in time over successive surveys. Using contrasts defined for calibrated beams means that performance standards (i.e. threshold contrast–detail detectability curves) can be independent of test object. The disadvantage of this geometry is that many other factors can influence overall (system) imaging performance and these are not assessed.

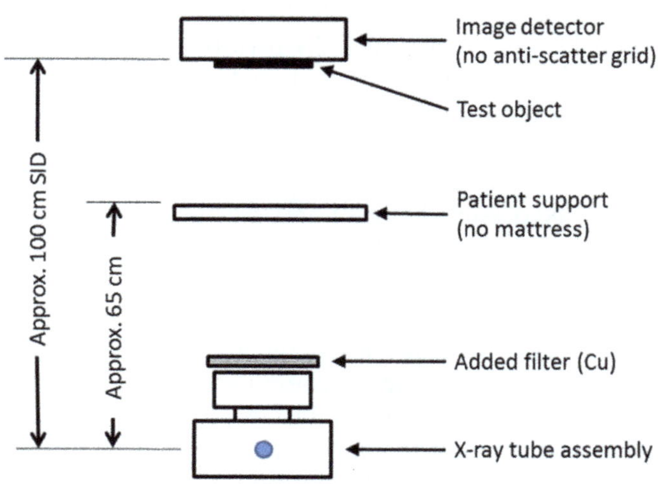

Figure 4.1. Geometric set-up for image detector based evaluations.

4.2.2 System-based technical image quality evaluation

In order to try and make a full system test of technical image quality, images of test objects are captured with patient equivalent attenuation, in an approximately patient equivalent position (with the test object at the isocentre, on the patient couch). This geometry includes factors such as the influence of the geometry (magnification), x-ray tube (focus size, pulse length), contrast (i.e. the selected energy/tube voltage), anti-scatter grid/air gap, and the x-ray detector, on the image quality measurement. This geometry certainly offers a more complete evaluation of the many factors that affect image quality, however, there are also some difficulties. There will be a wider range in geometries and these will depend on system type or application (i.e. a common geometry cannot be set) making large scale cross comparisons difficult (figure 4.2).

There can also be difficulties associated with obtaining a meaningful, generally applicable test object score, given the potentially wide range in energy/tube voltage used and the presence of scattered radiation. Essentially, the thickness, diameter, and composition of targets within the test object must be known if a universal or transparent image quality standard is to be set. Alternatively, if the test object composition is not known, then physicists would have to use the same test object if they wish to compare image quality results.

4.2.3 Static and dynamic test objects

Dynamic imaging image frames vary from the almost static scenes of the gastro-intestinal tract to highly dynamic image sequences of the heart. Because these systems provide live feedback on the region of anatomy being captured, the dynamic content of these image sequences varies greatly. Modern dynamic imaging systems

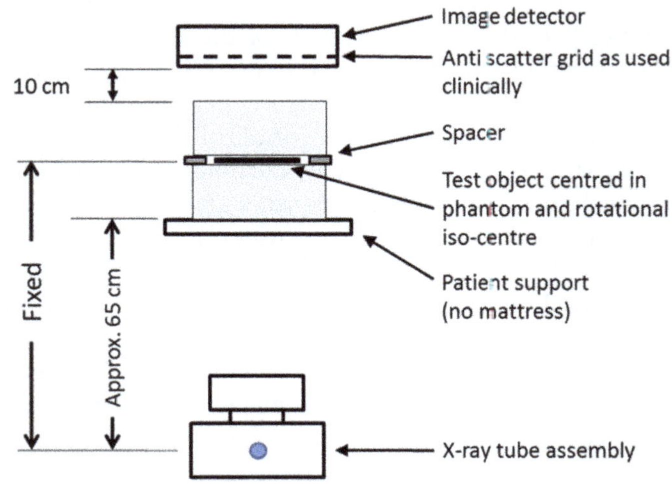

Figure 4.2. Example of the typical geometric set-up for a system-based evaluation (TO at patient equivalent position, scattered radiation, clinical magnification, includes source and detector blurring). Distances shown can be varied as required to simulate the clinical system use.

often use flexible recursive filtering coupled with motion detection algorithms that can be adapted or optimised to the degree of motion present in the scene being examined. Use of common quality control test objects (such as the Leeds test objects [1] or the PTW NORMI 4 FLU) can produce an overestimation of the image quality in the presence of recursive filtering algorithms, due to their static nature and the automatic averaging of previous frames in the run [11]. Therefore, while these test objects have been successfully used for routine quality assurance testing in the past, this type of evaluation strictly applies to image runs containing little or no motion, and in the absence of these types of algorithms.

Lag is defined as a signal that is present in the current image that was acquired for a previous image [12]; this can be a result of the delayed release of signal which then appears in later frames. We have to distinguish between two types of lag. First, many components in the fluoroscopy imaging chain will have an intrinsic temporal response, which will generally be signal level dependent (i.e. depend on radiation exposure). Second, recursive filtering, which can be considered as programmable lag, can be used to control the degree of stochastic noise present in an image.

One could make a direct assessment of total system lag (detector/camera lag and any applied recursive filtering) if the correct image types are available (see chapter 5). The temporal response will influence the technical image quality assessment made by using test objects. To assess this, test objects with moving components are required, in particular for cardiac imaging, where the linear velocity of cardiac arteries is typically 40 mm s^{-1} but can reach 90 mm s^{-1} [13]. While lag can cause blurring of objects that move within the radiation field during the time taken to acquire an individual frame, it can also be used to improve the signal to noise ratio (SNR) for static scenes and hence improve the minimum perceived threshold contrast [11]. Test objects developed to assess lag and recursive filtering include variations of the rotating wheel method that utilise the spokes to assess lag [14], holes punched in a copper plate [15], or a moving slit [16]. Other methods include photomultipliers coupled to a shutter [17], direct measurement of the (temporal) impulse response function [12], and rotating bar pattern phantoms [18]. A test object free method based on the temporal correlation of variance between frames has also been described [11]. The temporal sampling rate for all of these methods is determined by the video frame rate (f_v) and therefore is vulnerable to aliasing if the temporal response function contains frequency components above $f_v/2$. To overcome this, a method using a moving slanted edge that provides an assessment of the full pre-sampled temporal MTF has been described [19]. Another vital aspect of system performance, particularly relevant to cardiac applications, where rapidly moving objects have to be imaged, is the x-ray pulse length. The duration of the x-ray pulse determines the effective source size and hence geometric blurring for a given object [20]. As with focus size, the degree of motion-related unsharpness due to the source increases as the object approaches the x-ray source.

Standard detector geometries will not characterise this source of unsharpness. Guibelalde *et al* [21] demonstrated that increasing pulse length from 3 ms to 10 ms caused a significant reduction in contrast and SNR on a rotating spoke test object. This would suggest that tests for cardiac imaging systems should be based around a test object placed at the clinical position, using a test object moving at clinically realistic velocities. The current generation of cardiac x-ray systems try keeping the pulse length below 10 ms, even for patient equivalent thicknesses above 30 cm of PMMA. For example, figure 4.3 shows that a Siemens Artis Q keeps the pulse length at 3.5 ms up to 20 cm PMMA, pulse length then increases to 5.3 ms for PMMA thicknesses up to 27 cm.

4.2.4 Test object composition

In order to measure low contrast detectability, test objects produce small attenuation differences, typically as a function of size. A wide range of material composition and thickness is used. For example, the CDDISC (Artinis Medical Systems, Netherlands) consists of circular holes (i.e. air contrast) of different depths ranging in diameter from 0.3 to 8.0 mm drilled into a PMMA disc. The ACR Radiography Fluoroscopy Accreditation Phantom (Model 07–903) has 9.5 mm diameter holes of different depths drilled into a 2.0 mm thick aluminium sheet. A similar approach is used in the CDRH test object (Model 07–649), where the image quality test object consists of 9.5 mm diameter holes of different depths drilled into an 8.6 mm thick plastic disk (for high contrasts) and a 6.4 mm thick aluminium disc (for low contrasts). These last two test objects only provide a threshold contrast result for one detail diameter, rather than a full contrast–detail (*c–d*) curve. The Leeds *c–d* test objects contain aluminium, copper, and lead discs, of unspecified thickness, ranging in diameter from 0.25 mm to 11.1 mm, arranged on PMMA plates. All of these test objects make the assumption that the radiographic contrasts generated by these materials have a similar energy dependence to that of the anatomy of interest, over the diagnostic energy range, which may not be the case.

For clinical tasks where the anatomy produces insufficient radiographic contrast, contrast media are used in order to render visible the organs or blood vessels of interest.

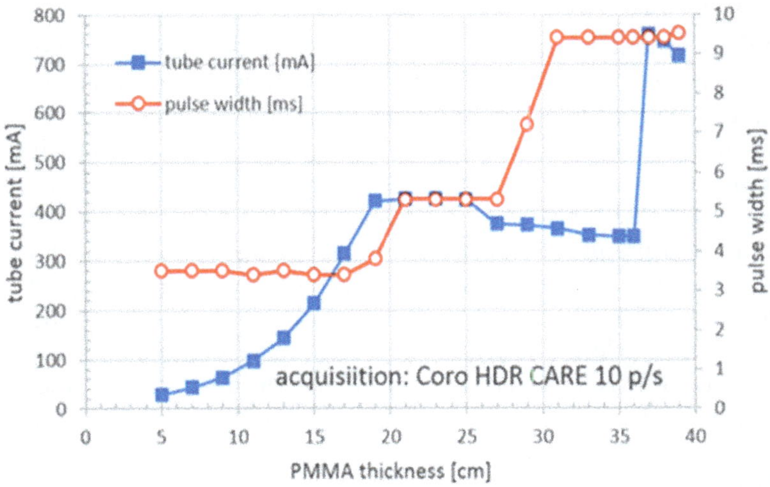

Figure 4.3. Peak tube current and x-ray pulse length as a function of PMMA thickness.

Contrast media generally contain elements of high atomic number, usually iodine or barium based, and generate large attenuation differences. The exception to this is the use of air or carbon dioxide to provide negative contrast in double contrast barium examinations. Given the presence of K-edges in the linear attenuation curves of iodine and barium (33.2 keV and 37.4 keV, respectively), combined with specific or tuned ADRC kV/mA curves designed to image these contrast media, some test objects contain inserts or discs composed of iodine [22]. An example of this includes the NEMA XR21-2000 Cardiology phantom [23] which contains holes ranging in diameter from 1 to 4 mm, filled with iodine of concentration between 2.5 mg cm^{-2} and 20 mg cm^{-2}.

There are test objects designed to test DSA modes that do not contain iodine-based targets. Similar to the Leeds TO10 fluoroscopy test object, the Leeds TO20 *c–d* test object [2, 3] is constructed from aluminium, copper, and lead discs, but the discs are thinner (i.e. lower radiographic contrast) than those in TO10 and hence can quantify the superior low contrast detectability of DSA systems. IEC standard 61 223-3-3 [24] described a set of test objects for the performance testing of DSA systems. This standard has now been withdrawn but test objects based on the standard are still commercially available, (i.e. X-Check DSA test object (PTW), QUART DSA phantom (QUART)). The test object has a 57 mm thick PMMA body with a 10 mm slot for a 9.5 mm thick PMMA slider. This slider contains aluminium strips 10 mm in diameter that range in thickness from 0.05 mm to 0.4 mm, simulating iodine contrast concentration of 5 to 10 mg ml^{-1} for vascular diameters of 1 to 4 mm. The test object also contains an eight step wedge composed of copper, with steps that range in thickness from 0.2 to 1.4 mm copper, to test dynamic range and the logarithmic look-up table (LUT) applied during DSA image acquisition. The Leeds test objects have linear and logarithmic step wedges for testing the accuracy and reproducibility of DSA system look-up tables.

4.2.5 Future developments

The technology behind dynamic imaging systems and associated sub-systems such as the ADRC does not stand still and there will certainly be developments coming in the future. This will include improvements in component hardware. For example, the implementation of flat emitters for the x-ray tube leads to foci with a square, consistent shape and therefore improved image quality, with isotropic sharpness across the image. The tubes have increased power and therefore smaller foci and higher amounts of pre-filtration can be used, meaning that the same image quality can be produced at lower doses. X-ray detectors with active pixel gain have been introduced, with lower levels of electronic noise and these may be useful for procedures such as electro-physiology, where very long fluoroscopy times are common and DAKR is kept very low (in the region of ~10 nGy/frame).

There will also be developments in image processing resulting from improvements in computing power and this will influence ADRC design. These systems will analyse the content of the image and adjust acquisition and processing parameters to maximise the visibility of 'clinically relevant structures' and diminish structures or textures considered to be noise. This is therefore a content-aware ADRC, using scene recognition techniques such as those used in digital photography. The clinically relevant targets will obviously depend on the task and this is of great importance for image quality evaluation; such systems cannot be evaluated using homogeneous test objects containing simple patterns. The ADRC will respond differently to (simple) test objects compared to clinical scenes and thus evaluation using an array of discs on a homogeneous background is likely to be of limited value. This also has implications for comparisons made between imaging systems—the hardware may be similar (x-ray tube, detector, etc) but differences in the ADRC could lead to strong differences in measured system performance—and these differences could depend on the test object used for the comparison [25]. Thus, the results of performance comparisons (image quality and dose) between different imaging systems (even set up or designed for similar clinical tasks) will require careful interpretation. In the long run, physicists will have to turn to more realistic test objects and develop techniques such as model observers to assess these test objects. These test objects will certainly not match the case variability or range of real tasks performed on interventional systems for example, but a simple, realistic task in a realistic background may give a more relevant/reproducible assessment of image quality than a low contrast detectability measurement in a homogeneous background. Model observers, either in the form a non-prewhitened (NPW) matched filter [26] or using channelised Hotelling observers (CHO), have been already been implemented as a means of evaluating simple test object based stimuli [27–29]. A basic computer scoring method has already been implemented by Leeds test objects in the form of AutoPIA.

4.2.6 Programme choice, test order, and geometry

Before providing detailed descriptions of each test, some comments on programme set-up and system geometry are given below. Over the years there have been different approaches in terms of technical image quality testing:

1. Image detector geometry at fixed energy and DAKR, i.e. set fixed imaging conditions with low scatter (metal) filtration and compare results against an absolute standard for the detector type. This method allows tracking of detector performance over time.
2. Clinical geometry, clinical energy, DAKR, and scatter phantom (the opposite of approach 1). If there is a reference curve for this type of measurement, this will relate to an examination (e.g. for the fluoroscopy mode used with cardiac imaging mode) and not a DAKR setting etc. Some interpretation of results is made, namely: is this level of quality appropriate for the tasks performed on the system? Provided the programme/settings remain unchanged, the system performance can be compared to baseline values.
3. Image detector geometry but with energy (tube voltage and filtration) within a specified range and clinical DAKR, low scatter (metal) filtration. This is a compromise approach to testing image detector performance, given the

difficulty in setting a specific energy and DAKR on modern systems. Provided the system is quantum noise limited, the image quality score can be corrected for differences in DAKR between measurement and reference.

Early testing protocols favoured the image detector/reference approach of the first method. Previous generations of dynamic imaging systems consisted of an x-ray intensifier system coupled to a TV camera (e.g. a Vidicon type). Typically, this had just one or two dose rate modes and the imaging performance of these two components could be assessed directly. It was generally possible to set a specific tube voltage and input air KERMA rate (70 kV with 1 mm copper and 0.26 μGy s^{-1} at the intensifier input face) (STB 7/82 DHSS 1982). The same factors could be set, the *c–d* curve could be derived reflecting the fundamental imaging performance of the intensifier–television system, and the curve could be tracked over time and compared to a reference curve acquired under these same conditions. This method did not explicitly evaluate the current clinical level of the image quality set.

The situation has changed dramatically over the years and the latest generation of dynamic imaging systems have imaging modes with a wide range of adjustable parameters that directly influence image quality as scored using test objects. It can be difficult to know all of the underlying parameters used in the measurement (e.g. pixel binning, target detector input air KERMA rate, spectral filtration, spatial and temporal image processing, etc). However, the programmes used for image quality evaluation must reflect the principal use of the system—in combination with a detector geometric set-up this is approach 3. It should be noted, however, that approach 3 can lead to difficulties in tracking performance over time; if the clinical use of the system changes then so does the common clinical programme and possibly the image quality. One option is to create a physics IQ mode with known settings (if possible equal to the clinical default) and use this to check image quality throughout the lifetime of the equipment. However, this will not represent the current technical image quality level as related to the clinical tasks performed on the system.

Given the widespread use of the Leeds test objects (originally described by Hay and Cowen [1–3]) by UK physicists, the description of detector testing in this protocol focuses on these test objects. This set of test objects contains phantoms suitable for assessing basic display greyscale, sharpness, *c–d* threshold detectability, detector distortion, FOV, and regional blurring. However, other test objects that provide similar information on system component performance can also be used. The Leeds test objects are calibrated for specific, low scatter beam qualities so that the radiation contrasts are known to a reasonable degree of accuracy. Tube voltage must lie between 65 and 80 kV for the programme chosen for image quality. Should tube voltage be greater than 80 kV then the copper filtration should be reduced (to 1.5 or 1.0 mm). If still outside the range (less than 65 kV with 2.0 mm copper in the beam, or greater than 80 kV with 1.0 mm copper) then use a different programme setting if available, although it is unusual to have to do this. One option to increase tube voltage is to add low atomic number attenuation such as PMMA, placed at the *x*-ray tube exit port to reduce the influence of scattered radiation on the contrasts.

The image quality tests can be combined with the ADRC tests in order to achieve an efficient set of image quality tests. A typical test order might be as follows:

1. Discuss the use of the system with the operators or even better an MDT (see section 2.4.3) in order to find out the clinical tasks for which the system is currently used, along with the most commonly used fluoroscopy and acquisition programmes/modes.
2. The settings of important system parameters (i.e. parameters that influence image quality and dose) are then recorded for these selected (frequently used) programmes. Note that the XR-27 User Quality Control Mode includes methods that document the system configuration such that the system protocol settings and any changes can be tracked.
3. The x-ray tube and generator tests are then performed, along with radiation FOV measurement and KAP calibration tests. The DAKR using copper filtration at the x-ray tube is then measured. If the UQCM is available then the detector performance tests (detector response function, MTF, normalised NPS (NNPS), etc) can be performed at this point. If being assessed, then the technical image quality tests with test objects positioned at the detector can be made. Finally, the ESAKR measurements are performed, followed by the technical image quality tests made using a system geometric set-up.

4.3 Assessment of detector technical image quality using test objects

These are made with a detector set-up and hence the test objects are placed as close to the detector entrance plane as conveniently as is possible. For R/F table systems still in service the test object can be positioned in the film/CR cassette slot of the R/F II tower. Table 4.1 provides a section summary.

4.3.1 Subjective analysis and observer error

The patterns generated by these test objects require subjective evaluation by human observers and hence are subject to uncertainties associated with human reading. Error on the *c–d* data can be calculated using the data of Marshall or Launders [33, 34]. Ideally the *c–d* test objects should be scored by at least two observers. In fact, it is often useful or even essential to have two people testing systems where, for example, one person has to operate the foot pedal in the x-ray room near the patient table, while the other person is behind the console in the control room recording the system parameters used.

4.3.2 Viewing conditions

It is important that the influence of factors such as ambient lighting and reflections are minimised during image quality tests due to their negative effect on perceived image quality. The viewing distance adopted by the observers can also have a major impact on the *c–d* evaluation, in particular when widely varying FOVs are tested and compared. Kotre *et al* [35] described a method of keeping the visual bias of the observers constant over widely differing input field diameters. The *c–d* results are effectively normalised for FOV differences using a viewing distance related to the FOV; comparison could then be made to a common reference standard. However, the

Table 4.1. Technical image quality tests.

Section	Parameter	Evaluation/test object	Acceptability criteria
4.3.4	Display device set-up	Visual evaluation/ Leeds GS2	All steps in step wedge visible; circular details visible.
4.3.5	Fluoroscopy detector threshold contrast–detail detectability	Threshold contrast–detail curve/Leeds TO10, TO12, or TO20	Compare to reference data. *c–d* curve should lie within $\pm X\%$ of the baseline value, where X is at the MPE's discretion. Methods for comparison to baseline vary [30].
4.3.6	Acquisition (series or cardiac) detector threshold contrast–detail detectability	Threshold contrast–detail curve/Leeds TO12 or TO20	Compare to reference data. The *c–d* curve should lie within $\pm X\%$ of the baseline value, where X is at the MPE's discretion. Methods for comparison to the baseline vary [31].
4.3.7	Acquisition (DSA) detector threshold contrast–detail detectability	Threshold contrast–detail curve/Leeds TO12 or TO20	Compare to reference data. The *c–d* curve should lie within $\pm X\%$ of the baseline value, where X is at the MPE's discretion.
4.3.8	Fluoroscopy detector high contrast resolution	Limiting spatial resolution/line pair test object	Compare to reference data. High contrast resolution should lie within $\pm X\%$ of the baseline value, where X is at the MPE's discretion [32].
4.3.9	Acquisition detector high contrast resolution	Limiting spatial resolution/line pair test object	Compare to reference data. High contrast resolution should lie within $\pm X\%$ of the baseline value, where X is at the MPE's discretion [32].
4.3.10	IITV focus non-uniformity	Meshes/Leeds MS2, 3, 4, or similar	No areas of blurring should be visible.
4.3.11	System fluoroscopy threshold contrast–detail detectability	Threshold contrast–detail curve/Leeds TO12 or TO20	Compare to reference data for similar examination protocols. Expected to be within $\pm X\%$ of the baseline data, where X is at the MPE's discretion.
4.3.12	System fluoroscopy threshold contrast–detail detectability	Threshold contrast–detail curve/Leeds TO12 or TO20	Compare to reference data for similar examination protocols. Expected to be within $\pm X\%$ of the baseline data, where X is at the MPE's discretion.

Table 4.2. Suggested FOV and attenuator thickness for clinical examinations (copper for the detector-type tests, PMMA or other (approx.) tissue equivalent material for system-type tests).

Clinical exam	FOV (cm)	Cu (mm)	PMMA (cm)
Neuro	20–25	2.0 if possible, else 1.0 or 1.5	16
Cardiac	20–25	2.0 if possible, else 1.0 or 1.5	20, 25, 30
Abdomen	32–42	2.0 if possible, else 1.0 or 1.5	20
Orthopaedic	16–25	2.0 if possible, else 1.0 or 1.5	10, 15, 20

method makes some assumptions such as the brightness control under the fixed conditions is the same as the clinical operation, and that lag does not change between FOVs (i.e. is not signal level dependent). Alternatively, a variable viewing distance protocol can be used in order to minimise the visual bias on the *c–d* curve [34]. This method corrects for the relative difference in air KERMA between FOVs by assuming quantum noise limited operation. The influence of the FOV on the *c–d* curve can be corrected by normalising detail diameters for magnification [36].

4.3.3 Test object set-up/imaging conditions

Once the most commonly used fluoroscopy and acquisition clinical programmes/modes have been established then the FOV, copper thickness, and PMMA thickness have to be selected. These will be related to clinical modes chosen for testing. See table 4.2 for some relevant parameter settings that are suitable for routine testing. When deciding on the FOV, this should first of all be relevant and practical (consistent test object positioning is difficult in a small FOV). Other considerations include trying to standardise to allow cross-comparison between systems (e.g. close to 25 cm FOV) and FOVs for which reference data exist. At commissioning, a wider range of FOVs, thicknesses, and modes can be assessed. Once selected, it is important that the same settings are used for QC over the lifetime of the equipment. If the clinical examinations performed on the system change, then the set-up should also be changed and baselines adjusted accordingly.

Regarding copper thickness for the detector tests, if possible use 2.0 mm copper positioned at the x-ray tube. If the programmed tube voltage for acquisition lies outside the range 65 kV to 80 kV then adjust the copper filtration (1.0 or 1.5 mm), repeat fluoroscopy, and check the tube voltage programmed for acquisition. There is not an easy solution if the tube voltage is still outside the range of 65 kV to 80 kV—this means that the TO contrasts are not known for the spectrum used. For testing acquisition modes, one solution is to change the acquisition programme settings (if possible) to give 75 kV and allow the system to set the acquisition mAs (if possible).

4.3.4 Display device set-up

Aim: To ensure that the display brightness and contrast are set correctly and the display is not the limiting factor in the image quality tests,

Frequency: 12 monthly.

Remedial level: All ten steps of the step wedge and the circular contrast details should be visible.

Method:

1. The technical image quality tests follow on from the ADRC DAKR tests and the geometry should be maintained, e.g. SID = 100 cm.
2. Set the copper thickness at the x-ray tube exit port and the relevant clinical fluoroscopy mode. Place GS2 (see figure 4.4) at the detector input face and ensure the test object is at the centre of the image for all FOVs.
3. Set a low ambient light level with no reflections on the display such that the viewing conditions are not limiting the results.
4. Image the test object for all FOVs. Record the number of steps visible in the step wedge; there should be ten; failure to see this number indicates a fault (TV display, TV camera, or incorrect LUT). The circular low contrast details should be visible in the squares.
5. If the greyscale set-up is faulty then alter the brightness and contrast settings so that the greyscale and circles are correct, however, there is little or no control over this for the latest displays used with FP detectors. For TV displays with hardware control over contrast and brightness, turn the brightness and contrast down to minimal settings. Turn up the brightness until the blanking circle is just apparent; then increase the contrast until all the steps on GS2 are visible. If the greyscale cannot be set properly then there may be a problem with the TV monitor.

Note: The use of GS2 is a quick, practical check. A full physical evaluation of the display devices should be made using calibrated light meters and test patterns, such as those detailed in AAPM Report TG18.

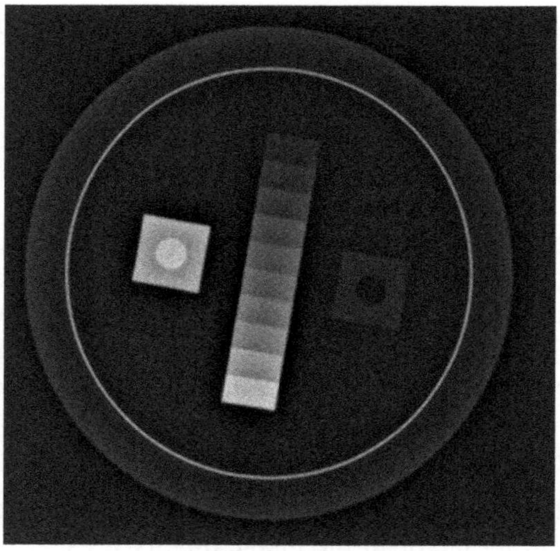

Figure 4.4. Image showing Leeds test object GS2.

4.3.5 Fluoroscopy detector threshold contrast–detail detectability

Aim: To assess threshold contrast–detail detectability of the x-ray detector.

Frequency: 12 monthly (extended testing at commissioning).

Reference curve: IPEM Evidence Base [31] or Evans *et al* [37].

Remedial level: Compare to the reference data. Expect *c–d* curve to lie within ±*X*% of the baseline value, where *X* is at the MPE's discretion [31].

Method:

1. Set the relevant FOV, copper thickness at the x-ray tube exit port and the fluoroscopy mode to be tested.
2. Place the *c–d* test object (e.g. Leeds TO10 or TO12) and ensure the TO is centred for all FOVs to be tested (refer to figure 4.1). Do not change the lighting/viewing conditions.
3. Record the tube voltage and mA(s), then count the number of discs that are visible for each detail diameter. For some programmes (e.g. GI barium-type) the tube voltage can lie outside the range of 65 kV to 80 kV, regardless of the copper thickness used. There is not an easy solution to this although in future it should become easier with the NEMA UQCM [38].
4. Use the variable viewing distance protocol [34] as this will minimise the visual bias. This entails using a longer distance for the larger discs while moving closer to the display for small details.
5. Score the images from live fluoroscopy, from the primary clinical displays (the main displays used in the room by the radiologist and radiographers). If available, the fluorostore function can be used when scoring the imaging. Maintain fluoroscopy for e.g. 10 s then press fluorostore and play back the fluoroscopy sequence ('loop fluoro' or similar function).
6. Repeat for selected FOVs. The current generation of FP based fluoroscopy systems can have many FOVs and there is little point in assessing all of these. For example, if a second fluoroscopy mode is often used then test this instead of rarely used FOVs.
7. *c–d* curves are available in the paper by Evans *et al* [37] for four FOV groups: 36 to 40 cm, 29 to 33 cm, 20 to 25 cm, and 16 to 17 cm (see table 4.2). These can be used as reference curves, but it is important to note that these curves were derived for IITV systems using continuous fluoroscopy modes.
8. *c–d* results can be corrected for differences in FOV used for the measurement and the reference curve: multiply the detail diameters by the magnification *m*, i.e. $m = FOV_{ref}/FOV_{meas}$.
9. If the contrast resolution of the system is known to be quantum noise limited then the *c–d* results can be corrected for differences in DAKR for the measurement and the reference curve: multiply the measured contrasts diameters by the ratio $(DAKR_{ref}/DAKR_{meas})^{0.5}$.
10. Error on the *c–d* fluoroscopy data can be calculated using [33, 34].
11. Also compare against baseline values to identify changes in detector performance (provided the same FOV and programme were assessed).

Notes

Unless there are suspected/known problems with the imaging system, one can generally assume that the system is set up to work in a quantum noise limited DAKR region. To determine whether a system is quantum noise limited for the imaging mode (e.g. fluoroscopy, coronary angiography, or series acquisition/DSA) the variance in the detector response function images should be examined as a function of DAKR. This requires access to For Processing images and manual control over the x-ray factors.

The figure of merit (FOM) proposed by Gallacher *et al* [36], calculated from the *c–d* curve and normalised for the influence of DAKR, radiation beam quality and corrected for pulsed fluoroscopy imaging (if used) can be used to track system performance over time.

4.3.6 Acquisition (un-subtracted) detector threshold contrast–detail detectability

Aim: To assess technical image quality via threshold contrast–detail diameter curve for (un-subtracted) acquisition mode.

Frequency: 12 monthly.

Reference value: *c–d* curve established at the commissioning tests, when the system has been configured for the clinical tasks performed on the system. Also see IPEM Evidence Base [30].

Remedial level: Investigate changes from baseline in the threshold contrast > *X*%, where *X* is at the MPE's discretion.

Method:

1. If measuring, follows on directly from fluoroscopy detector *c–d* measurement.
2. Set the relevant FOV, copper thickness at the x-ray tube exit port and the fluoroscopy mode to be tested.
3. Centre the TO12 or TO20 *c–d* test object at image detector input plane (refer to figure 4.5).
4. Perform a few seconds of fluoroscopy to obtain a stable image—this period of fluoroscopy is used by the system to programme the acquisition parameters for the acquisition mode.
5. Acquire the *c–d* TO images—this can either be at a slow rate (single shot or at a low frame rate, or at cardiac frame rates). For slow rates, acquire or evaluate at least two images per condition (FOV, acquisition mode, etc) in order to reduce the uncertainty on the observer *c–d* results.
6. For cardiac systems, set the commonly used clinical acquisition mode and acquire a sufficient number of frames such that a stable sequence is achieved (perhaps 8 s) and score using the cine-loop play-back function.
7. Record the tube voltage, mAs pulse length (ms), and pulse rate, then score the TO. As for fluoroscopy, use the variable viewing distance protocol when scoring the TO [33].

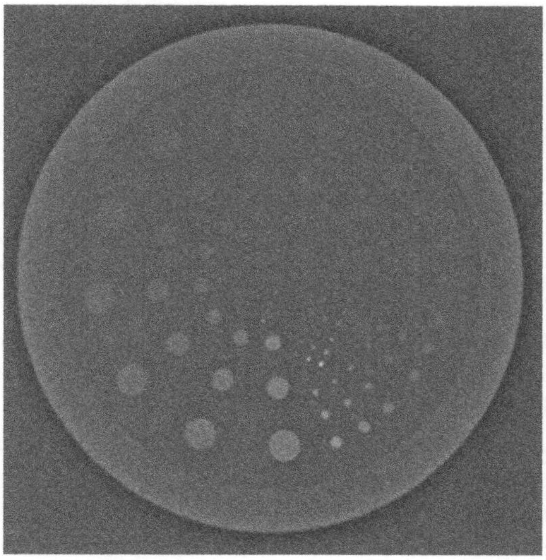

Figure 4.5. Image showing Leeds test object TO10.

Table 4.3. Threshold contrast–detail detectability curves from Evans *et al* [37] measured for well-adjusted IITV fluoroscopy systems (continuous fluoroscopy, low scatter, copper filtration, test object at the image detector).

FOV (cm):	16–17	20–25	29–33	36–40
DAKR (μGy/s):	0.70	0.48	0.27	0.22
[mm]	C%	C%	C%	C%
11.10	1.59	1.65	2.17	2.24
7.90	1.70	1.82	2.36	2.50
5.60	1.89	2.08	2.67	2.90
4.00	2.18	2.46	3.17	3.52
2.80	2.65	3.09	4.00	4.56
2.00	3.33	4.01	5.23	6.13
1.40	4.43	5.52	7.31	8.86
1.00	6.05	7.79	10.5	13.2
0.70	8.81	11.8	16.4	21.2
0.50	13.1	18.1	26.0	34.9
0.35	20.8	30.0	44.8	62.6

8. Repeat for other acquisition modes if used frequently on the system; test another FOV if relevant.
9. Compare against the reference *c–d* curve data for an appropriate acquisition mode if you have reference data. Some reference data are given in table 4.3.

10. Error on the static *c–d* data can be calculated using the data of Cohen *et al* [39]; error on the cine-loop *c–d* data can be estimated using the results of Marshall *et al* [33] or Launders *et al* [34].
11. Note that a higher DAK/image is used for acquisition modes (in the range 0.4 μGy to 0.8 μGy for iodine or barium contrast programmes) and hence these images may be structure noise limited to some extent [40, 41]. If this is the case then the *c–d* curve cannot be scaled and compared against *c–d* data acquired at a different DAK per image. Note that DSA sequences have (system) structure noise removed and can be scaled for dose/image, even if the DAK/image is high. When dose-correcting high frame rate (>5 fps) sequences (either fluoroscopy or cardiac acquisition) then we recommend the use of dose rate, i.e. DAKR. For slower scenes (<5 fps) (DSA or some native barium and iodine programmes), DAK/image for the dose scaling (if quantum limited) is recommended.
12. Also compare against baseline values to identify changes in detector performance (provided the same FOV and programme were assessed).

4.3.7 Acquisition (subtracted (DSA)) detector threshold contrast–detail detectability

Aim: To assess overall technical image quality via the threshold contrast–detail diameter curve for DSA imaging mode.

Frequency: 12 monthly.

Reference value: *c–d* curve established at the commissioning tests, when the system has been configured for the clinical tasks performed on the system.

Remedial level: Investigate changes from baseline in the threshold contrast > X%, where X is at the MPE's discretion.

Methods:

1. If performed, this test follows directly from the un-subtracted detector *c–d* measurement.
2. Set the relevant FOV, copper thickness at the x-ray tube port, and the DSA clinical exam to be assessed.
3. Perform a few seconds of fluoroscopy (obtain a stable image) with DSA programme selected so that the system can programme the DSA acquisition parameters.
4. Measuring the *c–d* performance for a DSA mode using TO20 is quite an involved procedure but can be performed routinely with practice. Prepare the subtraction test objects. Make two long tabs from paper tape (15 cm long) on opposite sides of the TO20 detail plate, similarly for the TO20 blank plate. This means that the TOs can be handled safely in the x-ray beam. For a typical image detector test geometry with an under table x-ray tube (figure 4.1), place the TO20 detail and blank plates in easily accessible positions on the table.
5. Hold and centre the TO20 blank plate at the image detector input plane (refer to figure 4.1) the paper tabs must be long enough so that hands/fingers are not in the x-ray beam. Start the DSA acquisition. Watch the display and

wait until the image of the TO20 blank disappears (subtracted) when this occurs the system has formed the mask image. The mask will be subtracted from subsequent images acquired during the run. Carefully remove the TO blank from the detector input, place the blank TO on the table, and pick up and hold the TO20 detail plate at the input plane such that its position is well aligned with the blank plate (this will be evident from the subtracted image). Maintain the DSA acquisition until a stable image of the TO20 detail plate is acquired, then stop the acquisition (release the exposure switch/pedal).

6. Record the tube voltage, mAs, pulse length (ms), and frame rate. Review the subtracted image sequence and select a frame in which the TO20 is stable (not moving) and clearly seen; score the test object.
7. Compare against reference *c–d* curve data for the DSA acquisition mode if you have reference data, otherwise look for baseline changes. The subtraction process removes detector structured noise and hence DSA images are not structure noise limited [41] (provided there is not substantial inter-frame jitter). Hence the *c–d* results can be corrected for differences between the measured and reference DAK/image levels: multiply the measured contrasts diameters by the ratio (DAK per image_ref/DAK per image_meas)$^{0.5}$.
8. Also compare against baseline values for this acquisition programme to identify changes in detector performance (provided the same FOV and programme were assessed). Some reference data are given in table 4.4.

Note

DSA is a very commonly used imaging mode on interventional angiography imaging systems and should be assessed.

4.3.8 Fluoroscopy mode detector high contrast resolution with a line pair test object

Aim: To assess high contrast limiting spatial resolution at the image centre and the ratio of centre to peripheral resolution and resolution non-uniformity for IITV systems.

Frequency: 12 monthly.

Reference value: IPEM report 91 (II detectors only) [32]. The evidence base shows that the typical resolution of FP detectors is much improved over these values. See EBQA publication [30] for updated values.

Remedial level: At the MPE's discretion [31]. The resolution should be in keeping with manufacturer-stated values.

Method:

1. Remove copper filtration and set the largest FOV, clinical default fluoroscopy mode.
2. Place the line pair TO at the detector plane to assess detector sharpness.
3. Ensure the TO is centred for all FOVs and orientated at 45° to the TV scan lines or FP pixel matrix.
4. The system should be selecting a low tube voltage under ADRC control, giving images with high contrast and low noise.

Table 4.4. Typical average threshold contrast–detail detectability curves measured for well-adjusted systems (low scatter, copper filtration, TO at the image detector, dynamic image sequence scored for cardiac programme).

Programme/mode	Cardiac acquisition	Un-subtracted acquisition	DSA
Average FOV (cm)	21	36	36
DAK at 15 fps (μGy/image)	0.09	0.67	1.74
DAKR (μGy/s)	1.31	72	69
Average tube voltage	67	72	69
mm	C%	C%	C%
11.10	1.70	1.37	0.41
7.90	1.78	1.49	0.55
5.60	1.90	1.69	0.72
4.00	2.16	2.03	0.99
2.80	2.64	2.60	1.43
2.00	3.40	3.48	2.11
1.40	4.74	5.02	3.32
1.00	6.91	7.48	5.30
0.70	11.0	12.1	9.07
0.50	18.1	20.1	15.6
0.35	32.9	36.6	29.1
0.25	61.5	68.0	54.2

5. Score the TO, counting the groups up to and including the last fully resolved group. This TO must be used with care given that most current fluoroscopy systems generate digital images and hence aliasing artefacts can be present [42]—stop at the first aliasing artefact.
6. Repeat for all field sizes.
7. Measure peripheral image sharpness for IITV systems as follows.
8. Set normal FOV and clinical default fluoroscopy mode.
9. Position and score the line pair TO at positions North, South, East, and West around the largest FOV. These results are used to calculate the focus non-uniformity and the ratio of peripheral resolution to centre resolution.
10. Peripheral resolution and resolution non-uniformity are not measured for FP detectors.
11. For analogue IITV systems, the sharpness is likely to be limited by the TV camera/system.
12. For digitised IITV systems, the sharpness is likely to be limited by either the digital matrix (large FOV) or the TV camera/system (small FOV): compare against IPEM report 91 remedial data or published national survey data [30] (see table 4.4).
13. For FP detectors, the line pair result is likely to be limited by the pixel spacing: the line pair result is expected to be limited by the Nyquist frequency for the pixel spacing $\mathrm{Ny}_{\mathrm{FOV}} = 1/2p_{\mathrm{FOV}}$ where p_{FOV} is the pixel

spacing (possibly binned) for the FOV. For line pair TOs captured at 45° to the pixel matrix then the Ny_{FOV} should be scaled by $2^{1/2}$.

14. Note: a measurement of the pre-sampled MTF offers a more robust quantification of detector sharpness properties (i.e. more repeatable and stronger correlation with perceived image sharpness).
15. Also compare against baseline values to identify changes in detector performance (provided the same FOV and programme were assessed).

4.3.9 Acquisition mode detector high contrast resolution with a line pair test object

Aim: To assess high contrast limiting spatial resolution at the image centre.

Frequency: 12 monthly for IITV systems, commissioning test for FPD.

Reference value: See EBQA data [30].

Remedial level: Compare EV BASED QA DATA. Expect to be within $\pm X\%$ of the baseline, where X is at the discretion of the MPE.

Method:

1. This test follows on immediately from the fluoroscopy mode measurements.
2. Remove copper filtration and set the largest FOV, clinical default acquisition mode.
3. Place the line pair TO at the detector plane to assess detector sharpness.
4. Ensure the TO is centred for all FOVs and orientated at 45° to the TV scan lines or FP pixel matrix. The system should be selecting a low tube voltage under ADRC control, giving images with high contrast and low noise.
5. Score the TO, counting the groups up to and including the last fully resolved group. This TO must be used with care given that most current fluoroscopy systems generate digital images and hence aliasing artefacts can be present (Albert *et al* [42])—stop at the first aliasing artefact.
6. Repeat for all FOVs.
7. Record the pixel matrix size versus FOV for fluoroscopy and acquisition; many systems display the pixel matrix as the FOV is changed. Alternatively, this can be done at the start of testing when recording the important system parameters. It may also be useful to check the pixel matrix and pixel spacing (e.g. DICOM tag 0018,1164 Imager Pixel Spacing: 0.154 0.154) in the DICOM header (required at the acceptance test). If doing this, then ensure that the sequences have not been down-sampled when sending to the PACS etc.
8. For analogue IITV systems, the sharpness is likely to be limited by the TV camera/system. For digitised IITV systems, the sharpness is likely to be limited by either the digital matrix (large FOV) or the TV camera/system (small FOV). Compare against data such as those published in the UK national survey [30], IPEM report 91 (table 4.5), or EBQA [30].
9. For FP detectors the line pair result is likely to be limited by the pixel spacing: the line pair result is expected to be limited by the Nyquist frequency for the pixel spacing $Ny_{FOV} = 1/2p_{FOV}$, where pFOV is the pixel

Table 4.5. Line pair TO performance data for IITV fluoroscopy systems from surveys and reports along with remedial level from IPEM report 91 (low scatter, TO at the image detector).

Source: FOV (cm)	TGR 32, report IV historical (lp/mm)	MDA report 98/68 (lp/mm)	IPEM report 91 (lp/mm)
40	0.91	0.84	0.69
35	0.98	0.91	0.75
30	1.07	1.01	0.84
25	1.19	1.14	0.94
20	1.35	1.32	1.10
15	1.58	1.60	1.33

spacing (possibly binned) for the FOV. For line pair TOs captured at 45° to the pixel matrix then the Ny_{FOV} should be scaled by $2^{1/2}$.

10. Note: a measurement of the pre-sampled MTF offers a more robust quantification of detector sharpness properties (i.e. more repeatable and stronger correlation with perceived image sharpness).
11. Also compare against baseline values to identify changes in detector performance (provided the same FOV and programme were assessed).

Notes

Detector binning can be different between acquisition and fluoroscopy modes. Definitely assess this at commissioning. If there is no difference between the results for fluoroscopy and acquisition, then just assess one of these modes (the mode with the lowest uncertainty on the result).

4.3.10 IITV focus non-uniformity

Aim: To quantify image intensifier distortion and focus uniformity using meshes.

Frequency: 12 monthly for IITV.

Remedial level: No areas or blurring should be visible.

Method:

1. Note that a visual assessment confirming the presence of distortion may be sufficient. If required, distortion can be quantified using the method below.
2. IITV systems only.
3. Set the largest FOV, clinical default fluoroscopy mode.
4. Centre MS4 at the image detector input plane.
5. Perform fluoroscopy briefly to obtain the LIH of the TO.
6. If the mesh is resolved then note any patches of poor focusing; if the mesh not resolved then change to a coarser value (M3 etc) and evaluate.
7. Repeat for all FOVs.
8. Alternative evaluation: calculate a variance image of the mesh using a 2 ×2 mm ROI. Note any regions of low variance (indicating blurring) and calculate the average variance for the FOV (and MS type).

4.3.11 Assessment of system threshold contrast–detail detectability

Aim: To track technical clinical image quality via threshold nominal contrast–detail diameter curve in fluoroscopy acquisition modes, including influence of scattered radiation, tube voltage, and source unsharpness

Frequency: 12 monthly.

Remedial level: Compare to reference data for similar examination protocols. Expected to be within $\pm X\%$ of the baseline data, where X is at the MPE's discretion.

Method: Set up the geometry for system testing, see the example for over couch detector and undercouch x-ray tube in figure 4.3.

1. Perform this test after making the ADRC assessment of ESAKR.
2. Set the FOV relevant for the examination protocol.
3. Place the patient equivalent phantom thickness relevant for the examination protocol (table 4.1) on the table. For C-arm type systems, adjust table height such that the object is at the isocentre (i.e. it should be possible to form typical clinical projections/views around the object). See figure 4.3 (section 4.2.2).
4. The *c–d* TO is positioned at the midpoint of the PMMA (10 cm PMMA tube-side, 10 cm detector-side)—centre the TO in the FOV before adding the remaining PMMA.
5. Start fluoroscopy and score the test object as described before (e.g. section 4.3.4).
6. Given the use of non-calibrated beam conditions for this TO, the contrasts cannot be calculated. One option is to convert the number of discs to a nominal contrast using beam data for 70 kV and 1 mm copper. This will generate a *c–d* curve that effectively plots the number of discs but allows standard c–*d* visualisation and a curve fit. Another option is simply to leave the result as a number of discs and track this in time (the total number of discs for the phantom or number of discs at a given disc diameter).
7. Record the source–test object distance (STD), tube voltage, mAs, and pulse length (ms), focus size set by the ADRC.
8. Compare against baseline values to identify changes in system performance (provided the same FOV and programme were assessed previously).
9. Repeat for the acquisition (un-subtracted) programme, e.g. cardiac acquisition
10. Repeat for DSA acquisition. For DSA it will be much easier to test as follows. Support the PMMA on small plastic blocks to (leave a ~3 cm gap between the PMMA block and table). Position the TO20 blank (or 1 cm thick PMMA) at the centre of the FOV. Start the DSA programme and once the mask image has been acquired pull or push the TO20 detail plate through into the centre of the FOV. Continue acquisition until the TO20 is centred and a good image has been acquired.

Note

This system test is expected to be more sensitive to changes in system programming (for example changes in focus size, spectral pre-filter, spectral energy) than positioning the test object and using the recommended calibrated TO beam.

4.3.12 Assessment of system high contrast resolution

Aim: To track system high contrast resolution, including the influence of scattered radiation, tube voltage, and source unsharpness.

Frequency: 12 monthly.

Remedial level: Compare to reference data for similar examination protocols. Expected to be within $\pm X\%$ of the baseline data, where X is at the MPE's discretion.

Method:

1. Place the patient equivalent phantom thickness relevant for the examination protocol (table 4.1) on the table. For C-arm type systems, adjust the table height such that the object is at the isocentre (i.e. it should be possible to form typical clinical projections/views around the object). See figure 4.3 (section 4.2.2).
2. The line pair TO is positioned at the midpoint of the PMMA (10 cm PMMA tube-side, 10 cm detector-side)—centre the TO in the FOV before adding the remaining PMMA.
3. Start fluoroscopy and score the test object as described before (e.g. section 4.3.4).
4. Position a line pair test object (or TOR.18) on the table and rotate such that the bars are at 45° to the TV lines or the FP detector matrix. The TO is therefore in a patient equivalent position plane, but is assessing the worst case for focus unsharpness.
5. Set the largest FOV and clinical default fluoroscopy.
6. Start fluoroscopy and score the test object.
7. Set low ambient light level and no reflections on the displays, as before.
8. Record the source–test object distance (STD), tube voltage, focus size, mAs, and pulse length (ms).
9. Repeat for FOV modes of interest.
10. Compare against baseline values to identify changes in system performance (provided the same FOV and programme were assessed previously).

This can be repeated for the clinical default un-subtracted acquisition programme.

References

[1] Hay G A, Clarke O F, Coleman N J and Cowen A R 1985 A set of x-ray test objects for quality control in television fluoroscopy *Br. J. Radiol.* **58** 335–44

[2] Cowen A R, Haywood J M, Workman A and Clarke O F 1987 A set of x-ray test objects for image quality control in digital subtraction fluorography. I: design considerations *Br. J. Radiol.* **60** 1001–9

[3] Cowen A R, Workman A, Haywood J M and Clarke O F 1987 A set of x-ray test objects for image quality control in digital subtraction fluorography. II: application and interpretation of results *Br. J. Radiol.* **60** 1011–8

[4] Suleiman O H, Antonsen R, Conway B J, McCrohan J, Rueter F and Slayton R 1992 Assessing patient exposure in fluoroscopy *Radiat. Prot. Dosimetry* **43** 251–2

[5] Siewerdsen J H and Jaffray D A 2000 Optimization of x-ray imaging geometry (with specific application to flat-panel cone-beam computed tomography) *Med. Phys.* **27** 1903–14

[6] Fetterly K A and Schueler B A 2007 Experimental evaluation of fiber-interspaced antiscatter grids for large patient imaging with digital x-ray systems *Phys. Med. Biol.* **52** 4863–80

[7] Barrett H H 1990 Objective assessment of image quality: effects of quantum noise and object variability *J. Opt. Soc. Am.* A **7** 1266–78

[8] ICRU 1996 Medical imaging— the assessment of image quality *ICRU Report* No. 54 Bethesda, MD

[9] The International Electrotechnical Commission 2003 Medical electrical equipment—characteristics of digital x-ray imaging devices—part 1: determination of the detective quantum efficiency *IEC Report* Geneva, Switzerland

[10] Mackenzie A, Doyle P and Neill J O 2010 Measurement of the performance characteristics of diagnostic x-ray systems: digital imaging systems *Institute of Physics and Engineering Report* No. 32

[11] Marshall N W and Kotre C J 2002 Measurement and correction of the effects of lag on contrast–detail test results in fluoroscopy *Phys. Med. Biol.* **47** 64–7

[12] Siewerdsen J H and Jaffray D A 1999 A ghost story: spatio-temporal response characteristics of an indirect-detection flat-panel imager *Med. Phys.* **26** 1624–41

[13] Lu B, Mao S S, Zhuang N, Bakhsheshi H, Yamamoto H, Takasu J, Liu S C and Budoff M J 2001 Coronary artery motion during the cardiac cycle and optimal ECG triggering for coronary artery imaging *Invest. Radiol.* **36** 250–6

[14] Moore R J 1984 Rotatable spoke fluoroscopic test object *Proc. SPIE, Medical Imaging and Instrumentation '84, (28 August 1984)* **0486**

[15] Shearer D R and Moore M M 1986 Lag in radiographic imaging systems: simple methods for evaluation *Radiology* **159** 259–63

[16] Okkalides D P and Raptou P D 1993 Quantification of image persistence in a digital angiography system *Br. J. Radiol.* **66** 882–5

[17] Gray J E, Stears J G, Lopez F and Wondrow M A 1984 Fluoroscopic imaging: quantitation of image lag or smearing *Radiology* **150** 563–7

[18] Rowlands J A 1984 Videofluorography: The role of temporal averaging *Med. Phys.* **11** 129–36

[19] Friedman S N and Cunningham I A 2009 A small-signal approach to temporal modulation transfer functions with exposure-rate dependence and its application to fluoroscopic detective quantum efficiency *Med. Phys.* **36** 3775–85

[20] Bernhardt P, Bätz L, Rührnschopf E-P and Hoheisel M 2005 Spatial frequency-dependent signal-to-noise ratio as a generalized measure of image quality *Proc. SPIE* 5745 407–18

[21] Guibelalde E, Vano E, Vaquero F and González L 2004 Influence of x-ray pulse parameters on the image quality for moving objects in digital cardiac imaging *Med. Phys.* **31** 2819–25

[22] Dehairs M, Bosmans H, Desmet W and Marshall N W 2017 Evaluation of automatic dose rate control for flat panel imaging using a spatial frequency domain figure of merit *Phys. Med. Biol.* **62** 6610–30

[23] Balter S 2001 A new tool for benchmarking cardiovascular fluoroscopes *Radiat. Prot. Dosimetry* **94** 161–6

[24] International Electrotechnical Commission 1996 Evaluation and routine testing in medical imaging departments—part 3.3: acceptance tests—imaging performance of x-ray equipment for digital subtraction angiography (DSA) *IEC Report* 61223-3-3:1996 Geneva, Switzerland

[25] Dehairs M, Bosmans H and Marshall N W 2019 Implementation of a spatio-temporal figure of merit for new automatic dose rate control regimes in dynamic x-ray imaging *Phys. Med. Biol.* **64** 045001

[26] Tapiovaara M J and Sandborg M 2004 How should low-contrast detail detectability be measured in fluoroscopy? *Med. Phys.* **31** 2564

[27] Favazza C P, Fetterly K A, Hangiandreou N J, Leng S and Schueler B A 2015 Implementation of a channelized Hotelling observer model to assess image quality of x-ray angiography systems *J. Med. Imag.* **2** 015503

[28] Bertolini M, Trojani V, Nitrosi A, Iori M and Sassatelli R 2019 Characterization of GE discovery IGS 740 angiography system by means of channelized Hotelling observer (CHO) *Phys. Med. Biol.* **64** 095002

[29] Villa R *et al* 2019 Model observers for low contrast detectability evaluation in dynamic angiography: a feasible approach *Phys. Med.* **64** 89–97

[30] Shaw D *et al* 2020 IPEM Topical Report: an evidence and risk assessment based analysis of the efficacy of quality assurance tests on fluoroscopy units—part II: image quality *Phys. Med. Biol.* **65** 225037

[31] Worrall M *et al* 2019 IPEM Topical Report: an evidence and risk assessment based analysis of the efficacy of quality assurance tests on fluoroscopy units-part I: dosimetry and safety *Phys. Med. Biol.* **64** 195011

[32] Hiles P A, Mackenzie A, Scally A and Wall B 2005 Recommended standards for the routine performance testing of diagnostic x-ray imaging systems *IPEM Report* 91 York, UK

[33] Marshall N W, Faulkner K, Kotre C J and Robson K 1992 Analysis of variations in contrast–detail measurements performed on image intensifier-television systems *Phys. Med. Biol.* **37** 2297–302

[34] Launders J H, McArdle S, Workman A and Cowen A 1995 Update on the recommended viewing protocol for FAXIL threshold contrast detail detectability test objects used in television fluoroscopy *Br. J. Radiol.* **68** 70–7

[35] Kotre C J, Marshall N W and Faulkner K 1992 An alternative approach to contrast–detail testing of *x*-ray image intensifier systems *Br. J. Radiol.* **65** 686–90

[36] Gallacher J, MacKenzie D J, Batchelor A, Lynch S and Saunders J 2003 Use of a quality index in threshold contrast detail detection measurements in television fluoroscopy *Br. J. Radiol.* **76** 464–72

[37] Evans D S 2004 Threshold contrast detail detectability curves for fluoroscopy and digital acquisition using modern image intensifier systems *Br. J. Radiol.* **77** 751–8

[38] NEMA 2018 X-ray equipment for interventional procedures user quality control mode *NEMA Standards Publication* XR 27–2013 (R2018) Rosslyn, VA

[39] Cohen G, McDaniel D L and Wagner L K 1984 Analysis of variations in contrast–detail experiments *Med. Phys.* **11** 469–73

[40] Ohara K, Doi K, Metz C E and Giger M L 1989 Investigation of basic imaging properties in digital radiography. 13. Effect of simple structured noise on the detectability of simulated stenotic lesions *Med. Phys.* **16** 14–21

[41] Marshall N W, Kotre C J, Robson K J and Lecomber A R 2001 Receptor dose in digital fluorography: a comparison between theory and practice *Phys. Med. Biol.* **46** 1283–96
[42] Albert M, Beideck D J, Bakic P R and Maidment A D A 2002 Aliasing effects in digital images of line-pair phantoms *Med. Phys.* **29** 1716–8

Chapter 5

Physical performance evaluation

This chapter describes the standard parameters used to characterise physical image quality, the appropriate use or scope of these parameters in a QC setting, and the steps required for their measurement in the x-ray room. A standard evaluation typically includes the response function (or characteristic curve), the pre-sampling MTF, NPS, and DQE. The focus is on the x-ray detector, however, the system sharpness can be assessed by positioning the MTF edge at a patient equivalent position. There is a large body of literature describing the theory [1] and measurement [2–4] of these parameters. Those unfamiliar with the theory and measurement should review the literature in order to understand the strengths and weaknesses of these methods before attempting measurements. A summary is provided in table 5.1.

Guidance for the characterisation of x-ray detectors used for dynamic imaging is available in the form of the International Electrotechnical Commission (IEC) protocol developed by medical device manufacturers [5]. Unsurprisingly, this protocol takes a similar form to earlier guidance on projection imaging for general radiography and mammography detectors [6, 7], but with an extensive addition dealing with detector lag. While the general principles of evaluation remain the same, the obvious difference when turning to dynamic imaging systems is that these systems generate dynamic sequences of images and the influence of the detector (or system) temporal transfer function (or lag) on signal and noise propagation must be accounted for if an accurate evaluation is to be made. Lag and the associated lag effect correction factor used to correct the NPS are discussed in section 5.7 of this chapter. Accurate, lab-based measurement of the lag corrected DQE of dynamic imagers, which can be used to benchmark and make comparisons between fluoroscopy detectors and systems, is not the aim of this section and is outside the scope of this work. However, an understanding of lag and its quantification is important and therefore the IEC lag correction method is discussed in this section as useful background.

doi:10.1088/978-0-7503-3819-6ch5

Table 5.1. Commissioning tests for quantitative analysis tests.

Section	Parameter	Evaluation	Expected relationship
5.1	Response function	Fit the model function; record R^2.	Simple relationship between PV and DAK; curve fit $R^2 \geqslant 0.99$.
5.2	Detector brightness uniformity	Max deviation on mean; inspect for artefacts.	Max deviation on mean < 10%; no significant artefacts.
5.3	Variance image	Examine variance image.	Uniform variance across the image; no artefacts visible.
5.4	Variance/noise separation	Fit (weighted) of linearised variance versus DAK/image; record fit parameters.	At typical DAK/image for each imaging mode, quantum noise should form the highest fraction of total image noise.
5.5	Normalised noise power spectrum (NNPS)	NNPS at 0.5 mm^{-1} and 2 mm^{-1} (or 1.5 mm^{-1} for a binned mode).	
5.6	Modulation transfer function (MTF)	Spatial frequency for 50% and 10% points of the MTF.	

Instead, the approach from IPEM report 32, part 7 [8] is adopted, with the focus on MTF and NPS as sufficient and valuable tools for tracking changes in detector or system performance. The DQE can be calculated but the limitations of the evaluation must be recognised. The exact measurement conditions for the NPS and MTF must be noted carefully for a given QC visit, in particular the applied recursive filtering.

5.1 Response function

Aim: To assess the output (in pixel values) of the x-ray detector as a function of air KERMA/image at the detector entrance, for the common imaging modes.

Frequency: 12 monthly.

Reference value: There should be a simple, monotonic relationship between the DAK/image and output pixel value.

Remedial level: $R^2 < 0.99$ [98].

The first step in physical image quality evaluation is the measurement of the detector response function (or 'conversion function', IEC [5]). This is established from a plot of the large area output level (pixel value (PV)) in the image versus the DAK/image at the detector surface plane. If working in terms of the IEC conversion function then the plot should be made versus the number of exposure quanta per unit area. This requires the definition of the beam quality for the evaluation and the air KERMA level at the x-ray detector for the evaluation. In order to be consistent with previous IPEM guidance on physical IQ measurements, we suggest a spectrum of 70 kV and 1 mm copper added, however, a standard IEC RQA-type spectrum could also be selected. Table 5.2 gives relevant information for these various beam qualities.

Regarding the DAK/image used for the assessment, the detectors used for dynamic imaging are likely to have three general air KERMA/image levels of operation, depending on the application: fluoroscopy, cardiac imaging, and series/DSA imaging. For these three exposure types, it is likely that the detector will be operated in a different gain mode. The IEC protocol defines the three imaging modes and associated 'normal' DAK/image levels, depending on the intended clinical use of the x-ray detector. These are 20 nGy/frame for 'fluoroscopy', 200 nGy/frame for 'cardiac imaging', and 2000 nGy/image for 'series exposures'. The DAK/image should be varied around the 'normal' level for the mode of interest—these should range from approximately a factor of 4 below the 'normal' level to a factor of 4 above this level. See table 5.3 for the DAK/frame range given in the IEC protocol. Note that these values/settings would be for a full evaluation of a given

Table 5.2. The IPEM radiation quality along with the RQA radiation qualities in the IEC standard 62220-1-3 [98] used for characterisation of diagnostic detectors. Shown is the HVL, the number of photons $mm^{-2}\ \mu Gy^{-1}$, and approximate mean energy.

Radiation quality	Approximate x-ray tube voltage (kV)	Additional filtration	Approx mean energy (keV)	Half value layer (mm Al)	Photons ($mm^{-2}\ \mu Gy^{-1}$) i.e. SNR_{in}^2
RQA 3	50	10.0 mm Al	40.3	4.0	21 759
RQA5	70	21.0 mm Al	53.3	7.1	30 174
RQA 7	90	30.0 mm Al	64.0	9.1	32 362
RQA 9	120	40.0 mm Al	77.0	11.5	31 077
IPEM 70	70	1.0 mm Cu	56.6	7.9 (approx)	32 300 (approx)
IPEM 70	70	2.0 mm Cu	60.1	9.0 (approx)	33 824 (approx)

Table 5.3. DAK/image levels and ranges for physical image quality evaluations depending on the imaging mode.

	Fluoroscopy (imaging mode 1)	Cardiac imaging (imaging mode 2)	Series imaging/DSA (imaging mode 3)
'Normal' level	20 nGy/image	200 nGy/image	2000 nGy/image
DAK/image range for detector response	0 (dark); 5 to 80 nGy/image	0 (dark); 50 to 800 nGy/image	0 (dark); 500 to 8000 nGy/image
DAK/image for NPS and lag	6 nGy, 20 nGy, and 64 nGy	60 nGy, 200 nGy, and 640 nGy	600 nGy, 2000 nGy, and 6400 nGy
DAK/image for MTF	64 nGy	640 nGy	6400 nGy
Total number of consecutive images	⩾ 128 (first 64 skipped, final 64 used for analysis)	⩾ 128 (first 64 skipped, final 64 used for analysis)	⩾ ~24 (first 12 skipped, final 12 used for analysis)

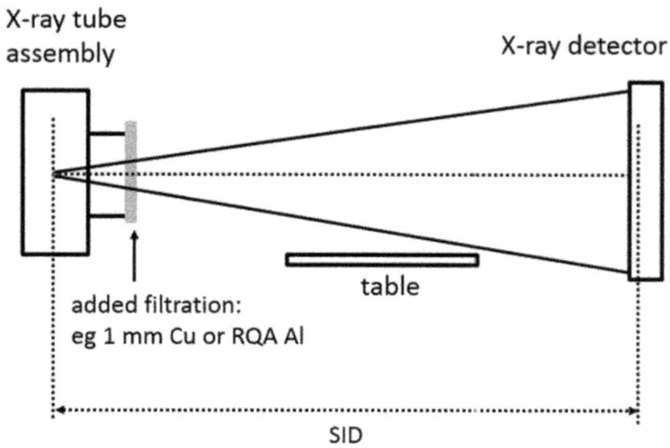

Figure 5.1. Geometry suitable for the response and NPS measurement for the physical image quality evaluation.

imaging mode following the IEC protocol—such a detailed evaluation is not required for an evaluation performed for QC purposes where a single (clinically relevant) DAK/image is evaluated. Regarding geometry, the response measurements could be made with a lateral set-up (see figure 5.1)—this allows easy positioning of the MTF edge later in the measurements.

Measurement of the response generally requires the use of manual control over both the tube and generator parameters and the detector/imaging mode. This can sometimes be achieved using an engineering/service mode that produces the required 'for processing' image types but will probably entail the use of UQCM made available by the NEMA XR27 standard. When acquiring a sequence of consecutive images at a given DAK/image for analysis, the sequence should include additional images (at the beginning of the sequence) that are not used in the analysis. The IEC [5] states that the number of consecutive images saved/used for a single DAK/image level (N_{IM}) should be a power of 2 and should be 64 or greater. The power of 2 requirement is related to the fact that an FFT based method (without zero padding) is used in the IEC protocol to estimate a factor that corrects for lag on the measured NPS (see section 5.7). For QC purposes this can be achieved when evaluating fluoroscopy and cardiac imaging modes, while fewer images should be used for series mode (which may operate at 2 frames/sec, for example). In all of these cases, an equal number of images (i.e. at least 64 for fluoroscopy and cardiac imaging) should be included at the start of the sequence that is not used in the analysis. This controls the influence of lag on the images used for analysis (figure 5.2).

If following IEC [5] then at each DAK/image level a sequence of unexposed offset (dark) images is acquired, i.e. x-ray beam off but detector operating, followed by a sequence of images with the x-ray beam on. This acquisition scheme is required in order to determine NPS for the dark images ($NPS_{dark}(u,v)$) defined in the IEC protocol [5]. Figure 5.2 indicates the dark and exposure images, along with the images to be discarded/used in the analysis. Note that adherence to the IEC protocol

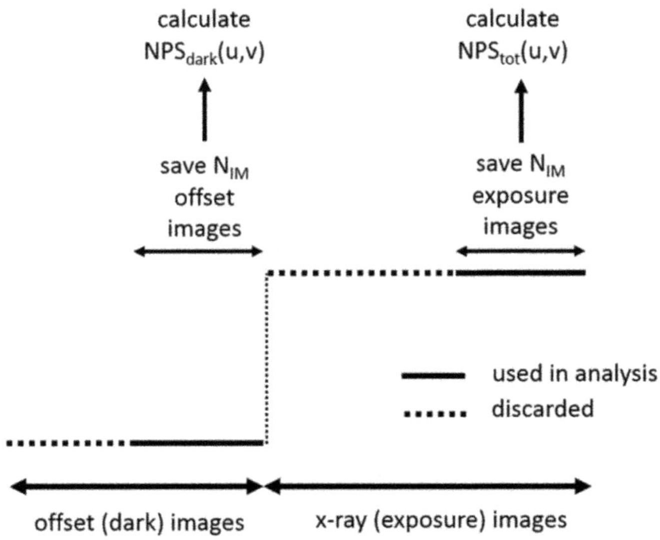

Figure 5.2. The IEC [5] acquisition scheme for the response function images, from which the $NPS_{dark}(u,v)$ and $NPS_{tot}(u,v)$ are calculated.

is not necessary for QC. Just exposure images can be acquired for a basic QC determination of the NPS but at least one sequence of dark images should be acquired, i.e. with the x-ray source blocked (under manual exposure factors).

Method:

1. Set a suitable mode for physical image quality measurements (manual, probably via UQCM).
2. Note the detector mode (fluoroscopy, cardiac, or series mode).
3. Set the geometry for the physical image quality measurements. Figure 5.1 shows a lateral arrangement suitable for the measurement of the detector response function and NNPS; this geometry allows easy positioning of the edge for the MTF measurement (see section 5.6). Alternatively, an under-couch x-ray tube with overcouch detector geometry could be used. While positioning of the edge at the detector is more difficult in this projection—this geometry would allow easy positioning of the edge on the table for measurement of a 'system' MTF, which includes the influence of focus size on the system MTF.
4. Set the beam quality for the evaluation, e.g. 70 kV and 1 mm additional copper.
5. Set the FOV, SID, and collimation to represent clinical practice; this may include the same SID as was used for DAKR measurements (see section 4.2).
6. Position the dosimeter on the axis, record the x-ray source to dosimeter distance, and calculate the inverse square correction to the detector input plane.
7. Remove the anti-scatter grid if possible.

8. Establish the tube current and pulse length settings required for the 'normal' level for the imaging mode and also to cover the DAK/image range (see table 5.2). If possible, maintain the tube current as fixed and vary the pulse length.
9. Remove the dosimeter.
10. At each DAK/image level (tube current and pulse length setting), acquire the required number of images (see table 5.2). If following the IEC [5] method of establishing the lag effect correction factor then at each DAK/image level, acquire a sequence of dark images followed by the exposure images (see figure 5.2).
11. Repeat until the DAK/image range is covered.
12. Measure the PV in an ROI of 100 × 100 pixels (or 5 × 5 mm) at the centre of the irradiated field.
13. Also record the variance of the PVs in this ROI.
14. Plot PV versus DAK/image (or Q photons mm^{-2}, if following IEC 62220-1-3 [5]) and fit the model function (typically linear, logarithmic or power—see IPEM report 32, part 7 for more information [8]). For example, versus K (DAK/image): $\text{PV} = A + B \times K$, $\text{PV} = A + B \times \exp(K)$, or $\text{PV} = A + B^C$.
15. Record the fit coefficients (A, B, C, etc) and the correlation coefficient for the curve fit (R^2) and track these over the lifetime of the x-ray detector.
16. From IEC 62220-1-3 [5], expect $R^2 \geqslant 0.99$ and that no individual data point in the response function deviates by more than 2% from the curve fit.
17. Repeat response function evaluation for the other imaging modes of interest.
18. The (homogeneous) images obtained for the response function are used for the calculation of the variance image, detector brightness uniformity, and the NPS.

5.2 Detector brightness uniformity

Aim: To assess the detector (signal or brightness) uniformity and check for the presence of artefacts.

Frequency: 12 monthly.

Reference value: Signal brightness should be uniform across the image; no artefacts visible.

Remedial level: Expect uniformity error < 10%.

Method:

1. A sequence obtained for the response function is used for the brightness uniformity calculation—see section 5.1 for the method used to acquire these images. Decide on the required detector mode (fluoroscopy, cardiac, or series mode).
2. Select the sequence that has a clinically relevant DAK/image and linearise the images using the response function for this mode. This DAK/image should be used for uniformity evaluation throughout the lifetime of the detector unless there is a large change in the set (target) DAK/image.

3. Go to the first analysis (x-ray exposure) image.
4. Calculate the brightness (PV) uniformity (see Marshall *et al* [9])—a typical ROI could be 10 × 10 mm. Record the coefficient of variation (standard deviation over the mean) and the maximum deviation of the central ROI.
5. Examine the image for signs of artefacts, in particular for signs of flat-fielding artefacts.

5.3 Variance image

Aim: To assess the global uniformity of the image noise power and check for the presence of artefacts.

Frequency: 12 monthly.

Reference value: Noise (variance) should be uniform across the image; no artefacts visible.

Method:

1. A sequence obtained for the response function is used for the variance image calculation—see section 5.1 for the method used to acquire these images. Decide on the required detector mode (fluoroscopy, cardiac, or series mode).
2. Select the sequence that has a clinically relevant DAK/image and linearise the images using the response function for this mode. This DAK/image should be used throughout the lifetime of the detector unless there is a large change in the set (target) DAK/image.
3. Go to the first analysis (x-ray exposure) image.
4. Calculate the variance image (see IPEM report 32, part 7 [8])—a typical ROI could be 2 × 2 mm, with half overlapping ROIs.
5. Examine the variance image for signs of artefacts, regions with reduced variance that could indicate blurring in the x-ray converter, and regions with increased variance that could indicate regions with increased electronic noise.

5.4 Noise separation using variance

Aim: To quantify the relative contribution of electronic (additive), quantum, and structure (multiplicative) noise sources to total noise (variance).

Frequency: 12 monthly.

Reference value: There should be a simple relationship between variance and DAKR; variance should be described by the three noise components.

Remedial level: At a typical DAK/image for each imaging mode, quantum noise should form the highest fraction of total image noise.

Method:

1. Use the variance data, measured as a function of DAK/image (step 13 during the response function measurement).
2. Linearise the variance using the response function [10] fit coefficients.
3. Plot variance as a function of DAK/image.
4. Fit a second-order polynomial curve to the variance, weighting the variance data points by the DAK/image when performing the curve fit. In this model,

total variance is the sum of variance due to electronic, quantum, and structure noise sources:

$$\sigma^2 = \sigma_e^2 + \sigma_q^2 + \sigma_s^2 \tag{5.1}$$

$$\sigma^2 = e + q\text{DAK} + s\text{DAK}^2. \tag{5.2}$$

5. If we express this function of DAK, the electronic noise (variance) coefficient is an offset, i.e. has no DAK dependency, quantum noise (variance) coefficient has a linear dependence on DAK, and structure noise (variance) coefficient has a squared dependence on DAK.
6. Record the fit coefficients for electronic (e), quantum (q), and structure noise (s) (variance)—track these coefficients over the lifetime of the x-ray detector.
7. Calculate the relative contribution of electronic, quantum, and structure noise as a fraction of total noise. Quantum noise should form the largest fraction of total image noise at the standard clinical DAK/image for the imaging mode tested.
    i. Electronic noise is dominant from a DAK/image given by e/q.
    ii. Structure noise is dominant from a DAK/image given by q/s.
8. Repeat the curve fitting for other imaging modes (fluoroscopy, cardiac imaging, and series imaging) if tested.

5.5 Noise power spectrum (NPS)

Aim: To assess the magnitude of noise power as a function of spatial frequency.

Frequency: 12 monthly.

Reference value: Record the NNPS at 0.5 mm^{-1} and 2 mm^{-1} (or 1.5 mm^{-1} for a binned mode).

Remedial level: NNPS at these frequencies should be within ±15% of the baseline value.

If following the IEC [5] lag effect correction method then see section 5.7 for information on establishing this factor and correcting the NPS. The lag corrected NPS is formed using the NPS calculated from offset (dark) images that is then added to the lag corrected quantum NPS. Note that the total NPS, calculated from the exposure images, could be used for QC purposes, provided some knowledge of the lag or applied filtering is known. This could just involve recording the temporal averaging (recursive filtering) applied to the acquisitions (for example, see the programme presets in the appendix). If the noise power is not corrected for temporal lag, then NNPS alone can be used, with no need for NPS (not normalised).

Method:

1. Set a suitable mode for physical image quality measurements (manual, probably via UQCM).
2. Note or set the required detector mode (fluoroscopy, cardiac, or series mode).

3. The images obtained for the response function are used for the NPS calculation—see section 5.1 for the method used to acquire these images and calculate the response function.
4. Use the exposure images to calculate $NPS_{tot}(u,v)$ at the chosen DAK/image—this DAK/image should match the value used clinically for the imaging mode. This DAK/image should be used for NPS evaluation throughout the lifetime of the detector unless there is a large change in the set (target) DAK/image.
5. At the commissioning stage consider assessing the NPS at the additional DAK levels, i.e. 1/3.2 and 3.2 times the normal value for the imaging mode chosen.
6. Normalise the NPS: divide by the mean (linearised pixel value)^2 of the region used for the NPS analysis (see IPEM report 32, part 7 [8]).
7. Record the NNPS at 0.5 mm^{-1} and 2 mm^{-1} (or 1.5 mm^{-1} for a binned mode).
8. Note that the NNPS calculated at this point is likely to be subject to the influence of lag that will reduce the NNPS compared to a measurement made without the presence of lag. This lag can originate just within the x-ray detector (specifically the x-ray converter layer) or may also include some form of applied post processing (frame averaging or recursive filtering). To establish the lag effect correction factor, see section 5.7.
9. Repeat the NNPS evaluation for the other imaging modes of interest.

5.6 Modulation transfer function (MTF)

Aim: To assess the sharpness of images produced by the x-ray detector (or x-ray system) using the pre-sampling MTF.

Frequency: 12 monthly.

Reference value: The MTF should correspond to a reference MTF provided by the manufacturer, for a given FOV and imaging mode. Record the spatial frequencies at which the MTF has fallen to 50% ($MTF_{0.5}$) and 10% ($MTF_{0.1}$) of MTF(0).

Remedial level: $MTF_{0.5}$ and $MTF_{0.1}$ should be within ± 0.2 mm^{-1} of the baseline value.

Method:

1. Set a suitable mode for physical image quality measurements (manual, probably via UQCM).
2. Note or set the required detector mode (fluoroscopy, cardiac, or series mode).
3. Set the geometry for the MTF measurements. The geometry in figure 5.3(a) allows easy positioning of the edge for the detector MTF measurement. Alternatively, an undercouch x-ray tube/overcouch detector geometry could be used (figure 5.3(b)). While positioning of the edge at the detector is more difficult in this projection, this geometry would allow easy positioning of the

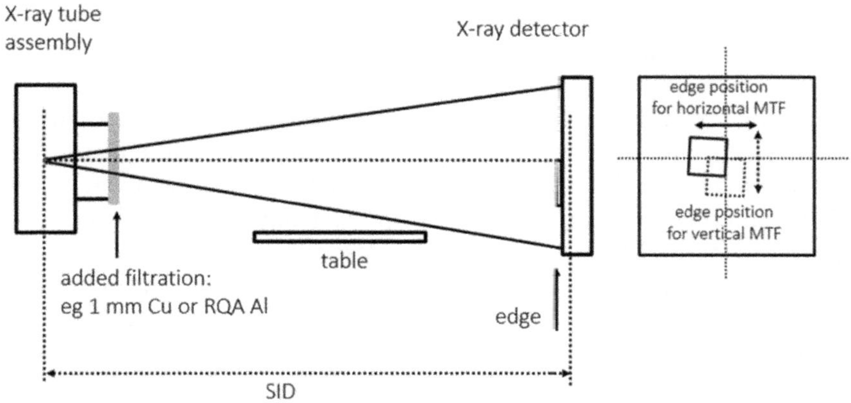

Figure 5.3. (a) Geometry suitable for measuring detector pre-sampling MTF. (b) Geometry suitable for measuring detector pre-sampling MTF and system pre-sampling modulation transfer function.

edge on the table for measurement of a 'system' MTF that includes the influence of focus size on the system MTF.

4. Set the beam quality for the evaluation, e.g. 70 kV and 1 mm additional copper.
5. Set the FOV, SID, and collimation settings to represent clinical practice; the SID may be the same as was used for DAKR measurements (see section 4.2).
6. Remove the anti-scatter grid if possible.
7. Set the tube current and pulse length settings required for MTF evaluation DAK/image level (table 5.2).
8. Position the edge test device to measure the horizontal or vertical MTF, as desired. Rotate the edge to give an angle of 1.5° to 3.0° between the edge and the pixel matrix columns or rows, as required.
9. Acquire the sequence of images.
10. Linearise the images containing the edge image using the response function (section 5.1).
11. Calculate the horizontal and vertical MTF curves (see IPEM report 32, part 7 [8]). It may be necessary to average a number of images before calculating the MTF, if the DAK/image is low (image noise is high), e.g. for fluoroscopy or cardiac imaging.
12. Record spatial frequencies for $MTF_{0.5}$ and $MTF_{0.1}$.
13. Repeat the evaluation for other imaging modes, as required.

5.7 Lag

An accurate estimate of the NPS and thus the DQE, requires an accurate estimate of lag that is present within the x-ray detector or imaging chain. Simply put, lag correlates the noise between successive frames, temporally averaging the noise; this in turn reduces the NPS and potentially inflates the DQE estimate. Higher lag could therefore be applied/engineered into the system or x-ray detector in order to bias the

NPS and DQE measurements; however, this would be at the expense of temporal resolution of the detector, obviously an important aspect of dynamic x-ray detector performance.

One means of quantifying lag is to assume that lag acts as a deterministic linear filter that is independent of DAK/frame and again use a correction factor that gives the NPS expected in the absence of lag [11, 12]. The lag correction given by Granfors *et al* [12] is found by operating the fluoroscopy system at the standard DAK/frame and the x-ray signal is then blocked. Detector readout is continued (not interrupted) for a period of time (frames) after the irradiation is blocked. The mean signal level at some ROI in the image is measured and normalised to a reference value taken from the images acquired with the x-ray signal present. This gives a factor used to correct the quantum part of the NPS. Friedman and Cunningham [13] describe the evaluation of the spatio-temporal MTF and DQE using a semi-transparent moving edge to estimate the small signal temporal MTF under approximately constant DAK/image conditions.

It is important to note that the detector lag processes within the phosphor or photoconductor only reduce the correlated component of the NPS, i.e. the primary quantum noise that scales with the MTF^2 and not the uncorrelated part [14]. Uncorrelated components of the NPS include additive electronic noise, noise aliasing, and secondary conversion noise. This is the reason why the lag correction factor [5, 12, 14] is only applied to the quantum NPS, i.e. ($\mathrm{NPS}_{\mathrm{tot}}$—$\mathrm{NPS}_{\mathrm{dark}}$). The NPS calculated from 'dark' (unexposed) images is assumed to contain only additive electronic noise that is not subject to detector lag. Of course image processing such as frame averaging or recursive filtering algorithms are applied once the final image is collected and corrected from the detector and these algorithms will influence the total (output image) NPS.

The lag correction factor described in detail here is that given in the IEC protocol for dynamic imaging [5], which in turn is based on the paper by Menser *et al* [15]. The method is extremely elegant. Just the steps required to calculate the correction factor are given—see IEC [5] or Menser *et al* [15] for greater detail. The correction factor is derived by comparing the variance of uncorrelated noise to the variance reduced by the lag in the detector. For uncorrelated noise, e.g. (σ^2_s), the power spectral density is constant, however, for exposed images detector lag introduces temporal correlation that reduces the variance (σ^2_g). The reduction of variance (noise power) due to correlation is given by σ^2_s/σ^2_g (figure 5.4). Given that the variance is the integral of the noise power spectrum, these parameters are derived by integrating the temporal NPS of the detector for uncorrelated noise and quantum noise ($P_{ss}(f_\mathrm{T})$ and $P_{gg}(f_\mathrm{T})$, respectively, in section 5.4)

Applying this method ideally requires programmable control over the x-ray source such that images can be acquired with and without (dark) x-ray irradiation. This is something that is difficult/not possible to achieve at a QC test, although an approach could be to use a beam block. The block should be positioned at the x-ray source and the relevant DAK/image set. Images are acquired in the desired mode and after N_{IM} offset (dark) images have been acquired, the block is removed and irradiation continued until the required number of exposure images has been acquired.

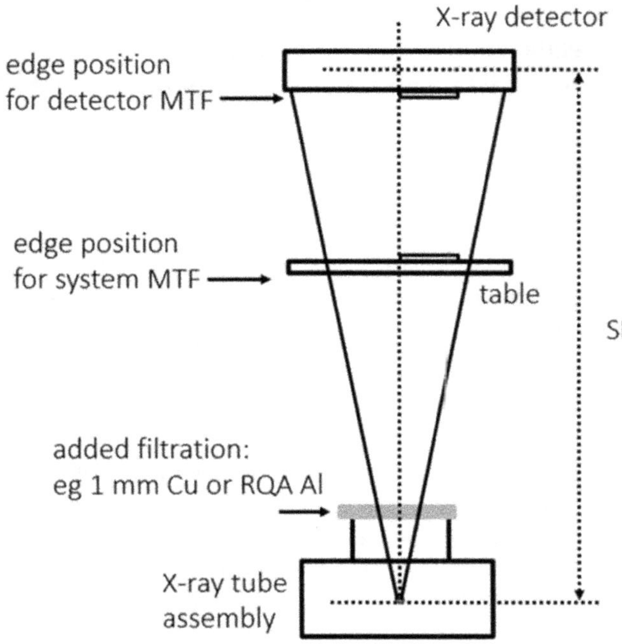

Figure 5.4. Power spectral density and variance of white noise (s) and correlated noise (g) as a function of temporal frequency. Power spectral density at zero frequency is equal for the correlated and uncorrelated processes. Variance is shown as the integral of the spectrum. The x-axis is the normalised temporal frequency, i.e. 0.5 is the Nyquist frequency [15].

Aim: To assess the lag correction factor required to correct the NPS estimate.

Frequency: 12 monthly.

Method: The lag correction factor is calculated from the same set of images used to estimate the NPS (section 5.4).

1. Select a central ROI that is at least 256 × 256 pixels in dimension in a given image for a given DAK/image sequence. This ROI is a set of K time signals $g_k(n)$ of length N_{im}, sampled at the frame rate used for acquisition, where N_{im} is the number of images in the acquired sequence ($N_{\text{im}} \geqslant 64$ and must be a power of 2). Increasing the number of pixels K in the sample reduces the variance on the averaged periodogram used to estimate lag correction factor.
2. For each given image in the sequence, calculate the average in the ROI (K) and subtract this for the ROI (K), i.e. the zero mean for each ROI in each frame.
3. For each pixel k within the ROI, estimate the power spectral density using the Fourier periodogram (i.e. fast Fourier transform (FFT) without zero padding):

$$\hat{P}_{gg,k}(f_{\text{T}}) = \frac{1}{N}\left|\sum_{n=1}^{N} g_k(n)\exp(-i2\pi f_{\text{T}} n)\right|^2, \tag{5.3}$$

where $g_k(n)$ is the grey level of pixel k in frame n, after subtracting the frame average. N is the number of images N_{IM}.

4. This results in K PSD results taken over the ROI (e.g. 256 × 256), which can be averaged:

$$\hat{P}_{gg}(f_{\mathrm{T}}) = \frac{1}{K}\sum_{k=1}^{K}\hat{P}_{gg,k}(f_{\mathrm{T}}). \tag{5.4}$$

5. The average of all the PSD is taken as an estimate of the *temporal* power spectrum of the x-ray detector. This is done for the x-ray blocked images to give the temporal power spectrum of the dark (offset) images ($P_{gg\_\mathrm{dark}}(f_{\mathrm{T}})$) and of the x-ray (signal) images ($P_{gg\_\mathrm{exp}}(f_{\mathrm{T}})$). Here f_{T} is the temporal frequency (not spatial frequency).
6. The temporal PSD of the exposed frames includes both (filtered) quantum noise (i.e. by the detector converter MTF) and electronic noise—however, only quantum noise is affected by lag. The x-ray and electronic noise are uncorrelated and thus the PSD for the quantum component can be found by subtracting the PSD for the dark frames from the PSD from the exposed frames. This gives an estimate of the PSD of the quantum noise that is correlated due to lag:

$$P_{gg}(f_{\mathrm{T}}) = P_{gg\_\mathrm{exp}}(f_{\mathrm{T}}) - P_{gg_{\mathrm{dark}}}(f_{\mathrm{T}}). \tag{5.5}$$

7. This has to be integrated to give the variance that has been reduced due to detector lag (σ_g^2).
8. As the average value of the data used for a PSD calculation has been subtracted, the value of the periodogram at zero temporal frequency ($P_{gg}(0)$) is approximately zero and therefore $P_{gg}(0)$ has to be determined separately. This is done as follows.
9. If the number of frames N_{IM} is sufficiently high, the PSD is oversampled and can be reconstructed from a subsampled version using $N_{\mathrm{IM}}/2$ samples.
10. Menser *et al* [15] showed that the unknown PSD at zero temporal frequency can be estimated as a weighted sum of the PSD subsampled at the odd positions:

$$P_{gg}(0) = 2\sum_{n=1}^{N_{\mathrm{IM}}} d\frac{N_{\mathrm{IM}}}{2}\left(\frac{2n-1}{N_{\mathrm{IM}}}\right)P_{gg}\left(\frac{2n-1}{N_{\mathrm{IM}}}\right) \tag{5.6}$$

where dN_{IM} is the Fourier transform of a modified version of the discrete rectangular window of even length N_{IM}, i.e. a sinc function:

$$d_{N_{\mathrm{IM}}}(f_{\mathrm{T}}) = \frac{1}{N_{\mathrm{IM}}}\frac{\sin(N_{\mathrm{IM}}\pi f_{\mathrm{T}})}{\sin(\pi f_{\mathrm{T}})}\cos\left(\pi f_{\mathrm{T}}\right). \tag{5.7}$$

11. The lag effect correction factor is calculated by taking the ratio of the PSD of the correlated (i.e. temporal low pass filtered quantum) noise to the PSD of the uncorrelated (i.e. electronic or dark) noise. The numerator is established by integrating equation (5.5) while the denominator is found by integrating equation (5.6):

$$r = \frac{\sigma_g^2}{\sigma_s^2} = \frac{\int P_{gg}(f_T)df_T}{\int P_{gg}(0)df_T}. \tag{5.8}$$

12. This gives the attenuation (reduction in variance) of quantum noise due to lag effects.
13. The final (total) lag corrected NPS is assembled from a sum of the dark noise NPS ($NPS_{dark}(u,v)$) and the lag corrected (re-scaled) quantum NPS ($NPS_{tot}(u,v)$—$NPS_{dark}(u,v)$):

$$NPS_{tot\_cor}(u, v) = NPS_{dark}(u, v) + \frac{NPS_{tot}(u, v) - NPS_{dark}(u, v)}{r}. \tag{5.9}$$

14. Note that the NNPS is not used for this step as this cannot be calculated for the dark noise NPS (there is zero x-ray signal).
15. If linearising using a response function of PV versus DAK/frame then the NPS is calculated from images linearised to fluctuations expressed in terms of air KERMA. After calculating NPS_{tot_cor} (u,v) then the NPS can be normalised if desired: divide by the mean (linearised pixel value)^2 of the region used for the NPS analysis (see report 32, part 7 [8]).
16. The 2D NNPS(u,v) (or NPS(u,v)) can be sectioned to form the 1D NNPS(u) or NNPS(v) (see IPEM report 32, part 7 [8]).
17. The lag corrected DQE can be calculated from

$$DQE_{cor}(u) = \frac{MTF^2(u)}{Q_{tot} NNPS_{tot\_cor}(u)}, \tag{5.10}$$

where Q_{tot} is the total number of photons mm^{-2} used to form the image. This can be calculated by multiplying the DAK/image by the number of photons μGy^{-1} mm^{-2} for the spectrum used (see IEC [5] or table 5.2).
18. If not measuring/applying the lag effect correction factor then DQE can be calculated as

$$DQE(u) = \frac{MTF^2(u)}{Q_{tot} NNPS_{tot}(u)}. \tag{5.11}$$

5.8 Example data

This section shows some sample results for a contemporary FPD based dynamic imaging system operated in fluoroscopy and cardiac modes. Imaging programmes were set with a linear look-up table, with no clinical image processing (edge enhancement, temporal (recursive) filtering, etc). The XR27 UQCM was not available on this system. The IEC lag effect correction factor was not evaluated. Figure 5.5 shows response functions measured using the IEC RQA5 beam quality. FOV was 22 cm for cardiac imaging mode and 22 cm and 42 cm for the fluoroscopy mode. The data show a linear relationship between PV and DAK, with $R^2 \geqslant 0.99$.

Figure 5.6(a) shows linearised variance measured in a 5 × 5 mm ROI at the image centre, plotted as a function of DAK/image (note a log–log axis is used). The fit results were: the electronic coefficient (e) was 3.90×10^{0}, the quantum coefficient (q) was 2.84×10^{-1}, and the structure coefficient (s) was 2.94×10^{-5}. From these coefficients, electronic noise would dominate from 13.8 nGy/frame and structure noise would dominate from 9642 μGy/frame. Note that these are only approximate figures—the key point is that, on the basis of image variance, quantum noise forms the largest component of total image noise over the typical DAK/frame used for cardiac imaging on this system (140 nGy/frame on this system) (see figure 5.6(b)). Also note that the magnitudes of these figures are specific to the system (and probably to the imaging mode and FOV used); absolute values for these coefficients must not be compared between different systems. The value of this analysis lies in uncovering the relationship between the different noise sources as a function of DAK/image.

Figure 5.7(a) shows the pre-sampling MTF measured for the horizontal and vertical directions across the detector, with the edge positioned at the (accessible) detector input plane. Data are shown for the FOV 22 cm and 42 cm FOVs; it can be

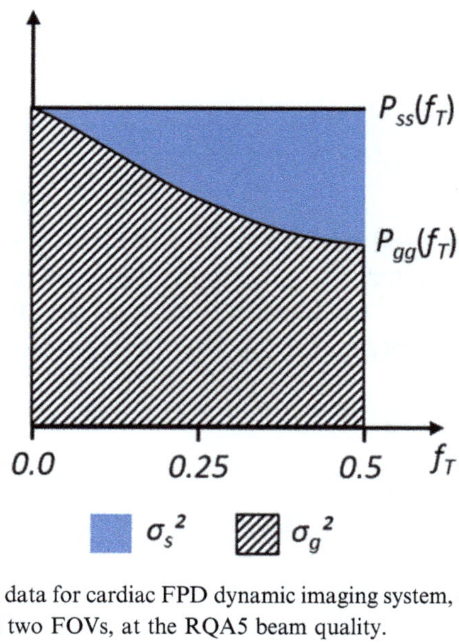

Figure 5.5. Response function data for cardiac FPD dynamic imaging system, operated in two imaging modes (fluoroscopy and cardiac) and two FOVs, at the RQA5 beam quality.

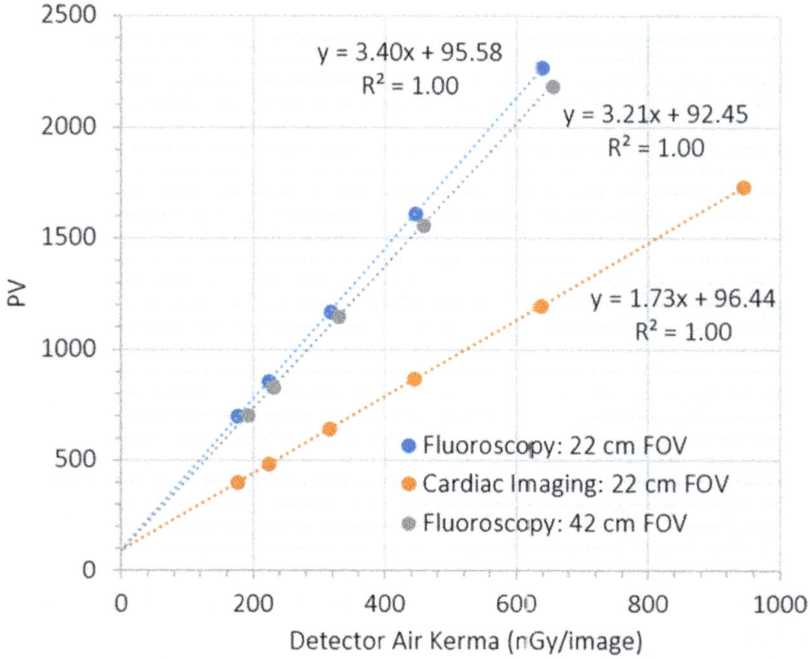

Figure 5.6. (a) Variance versus DAK/image and second-order polynomial curve fit, for 22 cm FOV, cardiac imaging mode. (b) Electronic, quantum, and structure variance expressed as a fraction of total noise, as a function of DAK/image.

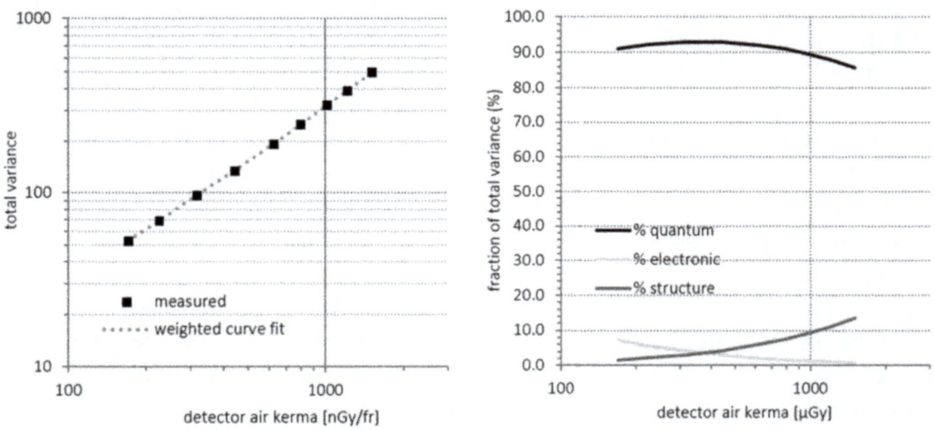

Figure 5.7. (a) Pre-sampling detector MTF measured for 22 cm FOV in the horizontal and vertical directions and for the 42 cm FOV (a binned mode). Edge positioned at the detector using the small focus. (b) Pre-sampling system MTF measured for 22 cm FOV in the horizontal direction (edge positioned at 70 cm from the source). Also shown is the detector MTF, measured with the edge at the detector.

seen that the 42 cm FOV is a binned pixel mode. Figure 5.7(b) shows MTF curves measured with the edge positioned at 70 cm from the source (approximate source–object distance), for three different focus sizes available on the system. This clearly shows the influence of extended source size (unsharpness) on the MTF, i.e. this is

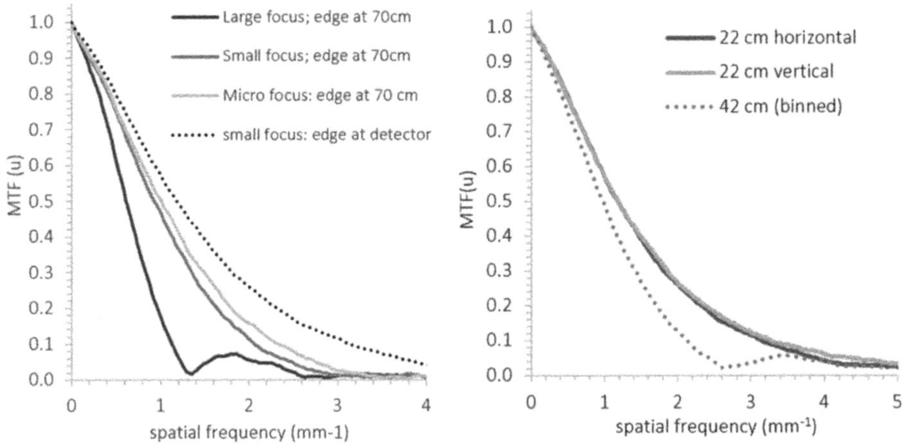

Figure 5.8. (a) Measured using the IEC RQA5 quality, for 22 cm FOV in cardiac imaging mode. (b) Radially averaged normalised noise power spectrum (NNPS). (c) Detective quantum efficiency (DQE), calculated from average pre-sampling MTF and radially average NNPS.

something like a 'system' MTF. The detector pixel spacing is 0.154 mm; 0.300 for the binned mode.

Figure 5.8(a) demonstrates a systematic reduction in $NNPS_{tot}$ as DAK/frame is increased, while figure 5.8(b) shows the resulting DQE curves. DQE is seen to be approximately constant as DAK/frame is changed, consistent with x-ray quantum noise being the dominant image noise source. These results are consistent with the noise separation (polynomial) curve fit data, expected as the NPS is the variance divided over spatial frequency channels. Some influence of structure noise at low spatial frequency (~0.25 mm^{-1}) is seen in the NNPS curve and this in turn leads to a reduction in DQE at low spatial frequencies. Note that this is the total NNPS (i.e. $NNPS_{tot}(u)$) and associated DQE—no estimation of the lag effect correction factor was made.

With the edge positioned at the x-ray detector input plane, then this type of evaluation is explicitly focused on the x-ray detector. The DQE measurements provide information on the efficiency of the x-ray detector that underpins the imaging system (and as such are crucial) but are just the starting point for the final (clinical) image quality presented to the operator. This would be tuned to the tasks performed on the system and many more parameters should be considered including tube voltage, pre-filtration, DAK/frame, frame rate, pulse length, focus size, geometric magnification, scattered radiation management, programmed temporal frame averaging, and the final clinical image processing set.

References

[1] Cunningham I A 2000 Applied linear-systems theory *Handbook of Medical Imaging Vol I: Medical Physics and Psychophysics* ed J Beutel, H Kundel and R Van Metter (Bellingham, WA: SPIE)

[2] Dobbins J T, Ergun D L, Rutz L, Hinshaw D A, Blume H and Clark D C 1995 DQE(*f*) of four generations of computed radiography acquisition devices *Med. Phys.* **22** 1581–93

[3] Samei E, Ranger N T, Dobbins J T and Chen Y 2006 Intercomparison of methods for image quality characterization. I. Modulation transfer function *Med. Phys.* **33** 1454–65

[4] Dobbins J T, Samei E, Ranger N T and Chen Y 2006 Intercomparison of methods for image quality characterization. II. Noise power spectrum *Med. Phys.* **33** 1466

[5] IEC 2008 Medical electrical equipment—characteristics of digital x-ray imaging devices—Part 1–3: determination of the detective quantum efficiency—detectors used in dynamic imaging *IEC Report* Geneva, Switzerland

[6] IEC 2003 Medical electrical equipment—characteristics of digital x-ray imaging devices—Part 1: determination of the detective quantum efficiency *IEC Report* Geneva, Switzerland

[7] IEC 2007 Medical electrical equipment—characteristics of digital x-ray imaging devices—Part 1–2: determination of the detective quantum efficiency—detectors used in mammography *IEC Report* Geneva, Switzerland

[8] Mackenzie A, Doyle P, Honey I, Marshall N, O'Neill J, Smail M, Dosh S and Hill A 2010 Measurement of the performance characteristics of diagnostic x-ray systems: digital imaging systems *IPEM Report* 32 (part 7) York, UK

[9] Marshall N W, Mackenzie A and Honey I D 2011 Quality control measurements for digital x-ray detectors *Phys. Med. Biol.* **56** 979

[10] Mackenzie A 2008 Validation of correction methods for the non-linear response of digital radiography systems *Br. J. Radiol.* **81** 341–5

[11] Siewerdsen J H and Jaffray D A 1999 A ghost story: spatio-temporal response characteristics of an indirect-detection flat-panel imager *Med. Phys.* **26** 1624–41

[12] Granfors P R, Aufrichtig R, Possin G E, Giambattista B W, Huang Z S, Liu J and Ma B 2003 Performance of a 41 × 41 cm^2 amorphous silicon flat panel x-ray detector designed for angiographic and R&F imaging applications *Med. Phys.* **30** 2715–26

[13] Friedman S N and Cunningham I A 2009 A small-signal approach to temporal modulation transfer functions with exposure-rate dependence and its application to fluoroscopic detective quantum efficiency *Med. Phys.* **36** 3775–85

[14] Akbarpour R, Friedman S N, Siewerdsen J H, Neary J D and Cunningham I A 2007 Signal and noise transfer in spatiotemporal quantum-based imaging systems *J. Opt. Soc. Am.* A **24** B151–64

[15] Menser M, Bastiaens B, Nascetti R J M, Overdick A and Simon M 2005 Linear system models for lag in flat dynamic x-ray detectors *Proc. SPIE* **5745** 430–41

Appendix A

A.1 Leeds test objects including TOR-CDR, TO10, TO12, TO20, TODR

Technical details can all be found at https://www.leedstestobjects.com/.

A.2 Calculation of uncertainty on the *c–d* curve

Cohen *et al* [1] described a method to establish the uncertainty on threshold contrasts measured by the observer for a particular contrast–detail curve reading. This method was later applied to dynamic sequences [2, 3]. Three sources of uncertainty are assumed: within-observer variance (S_{wo}), between-observer variance (S_{bo}), and case-sample variance (S_{c}). Within-observer variance arises from differences in an individual observer's decisions made on the same image sample over repeated reading sessions. Between-observer variance comes from differences in observer response (given the same stimulus) from observer to observer. The case-sample variance is due to differences in the mean difficulty of the observational task between two samples of the image data. These components are combined to give the relative standard deviation as follows:

$$\mathrm{SE} = \left(S_{\mathrm{c}}^2 + \frac{S_{\mathrm{bo}}^2}{l} + \frac{S_{\mathrm{wo}}^2}{lm} \right)^{1/2}, \tag{A.1}$$

where l is the number of (independent) observers, m is the number of times that the image (case-sample) is read. For a dynamic image sequences (fluoroscopy, cardiac series) S_{c} is assumed to be zero. For a single image, the data of Cohen (with S_{c}) should be used. Data for the parameters are given in table A.1.

A.3 Calculation of Gallacher IQ index

Gallacher *et al* describe a single, normalised IQ index (Q_{n}), calculated from *c–d* data, that can be used to track performance changes in fluoroscopy and acquisition *c–d*

Table A.1. Fractional standard deviations for use in equation (A.1).

Source of variation	S_{wo}	S_{bo}	S_c
Cohen *et al*	0.108	0.143	0.137
Launders *et al*	0.150	0.200	—
Marshall *et al*	0.115	0.111	—

performance over time. A reference *c–d* curve is chosen, for example the *c–d* data for the 20–25 cm FOV in Evans *et al.* The first step is to calculate Q, as the average of the ratio of detection index (H_T) for a given detail diameter to the detection index for the reference curve (H_{Tref}), for that detail:

$$Q = \frac{1}{n}\sum_{i=1}^{n}\frac{H_T(A_i)}{H_{Tref}(A_i)}. \tag{A.2}$$

The H_T index is defined as

$$H_T(A) = \frac{1}{C_T\sqrt{A}}, \tag{A.3}$$

where C_T is the measured threshold contrast (corrected for the beam quality used in the measurement, using the table in the Leeds TOs) for a disc of area A.

The Q index for the *c–d* data measured at a DAKR of K_m is then normalised for the DAKR of the reference curve, e.g. 480 nGy/s for the Evans *et al* 20–25 cm curve:

$$Q_n = Q\left(\frac{K_{ref}}{K_m}\right)^{1/2}. \tag{A.4}$$

A further correction factor for the change in II input phosphor absorption efficiency with beam quality (table A.2). This is required as the ratio of mass energy absorption coefficients of the caesium iodide (CsI) phosphor to air is not constant over the range of beam qualities used in the Leeds TO10 test object measurements. CsI is the scintillation phosphor in all current medical XRIIs and in all current medical FPDs used for fluoroscopy and angiography/DSA/cardio work.

Finally, a correction is made so the index can cover pulsed fluoroscopy systems. The correction factor is taken from the paper of Aufrichtig *et al* that describes the influence of image pulse rate on perceived contrast.

The final normalised IQ index is given by

$$Q_n = Q\left(\frac{P(f)K_{ref}}{R_n(V, X)K_m}\right)^{1/2}, \tag{A.5}$$

where K_m = measured input DAKR of the system in nGy/s, K_{ref} = input DAKR for the reference curve of the system in nGy/s, $R_n(V,X)$ = radiation beam quality normalised factor and is a function of V (tube voltage) and X (beam attenuation in mm copper), and $P(f)$ = pulsed fluoroscopy correction factor (see table A.3).

Table A.2. The ratio of mass energy $R(V, X)$ absorption coefficients for caesium iodide to air for different beam qualities (V = tube voltage, X = Cu (mm)), and normalised beam quality factor $R_n(V, X)$ to 70 kVp, 1 mm Cu.

Tube voltage (kV)	Cu filter (mm)	Spectrum mean energy (keV)	Ratio $R(V, X)$ of mass energy absorption coefficients (CsI to air)[a]	Normalised ratio $R_n(X, V)$ to 70 kV, 2.0 mm Cu
65	1	52.5	160.6	1.05
	1.5	54.5	159.3	1.04
	2	55.9	157.8	1.03
70	1	55.2	158.6	1.04
	1.5	57.5	155.5	1.02
	2	59.0	152.8	1.00
75	1	58.0	154.6	1.01
	1.5	60.4	149.9	0.99
	2	62.0	146.3	0.96
80	1	60.4	149.9	0.99
	1.5	62.9	144.1	0.95
	2	64.7	139.4	0.92

[a] For a 12° W anode, 0% ripple, 3 mm Al filtration.

Table A.3. Modifying factors for pulsed fluoroscopy ($P(f)$).

Pulse frequency (p/s)	Pulsed fluoroscopy equivalent perception dose modifying factor $P(f)$
30	1.00
15	0.78
10	0.62
7.5	0.51
3	0.19

Table A.4. Proposed fluoroscopy threshold *c–d* detectability criteria levels.

Classification	Q_n (dose normalised quality index) for fluoroscopy
Good	>1.2
Satisfactory	1.0–1.2
Marginal	0.8–1.0
Poor	<0.8

Gallacher *et al* give some levels which may be used to give an idea of overall system performance. As Gallacher *et al* stress, the Q index should not be used in isolation to other image quality performance metrics, for example the *c–d* curve itself, the sharpness results (MTF and/or line pair result), NPS, DQE, etc (table A.4).

References

[1] Cohen G, McDaniel D L and Wagner L K 1984 Analysis of variations in contrast-detail experiments *Med. Phys.* **11** 469–73

[2] Marshall N W, Faulkner K, Kotre C J and Robson K 1992 Analysis of variations in contrast-detail measurements performed on image intensifier-television systems *Phys. Med. Biol.* **37** 2297–302

[3] Launders J H, McArdle S, Workman A and Cowen A R 1995 Update on the recommended viewing protocol for FAXIL threshold contrast detail detectability test objects used in television fluoroscopy *Br. J. Radiol.* **68** 70–7

Glossary

ADRC	Automatic dose rate control: the negative feedback loop used to ensure dynamic constancy of image quality.
Acquisition	Automatic storage of a fluoroscopy run at a higher level of image quality (and therefore patient dose); this was referred to as 'cine' for IITV systems.
AGC	Automatic gain control; electronic gain applied to the displayed image to ensure adequate brightness.
ALARP	As low as reasonably practicable (achievable in some other countries).
CBCT	Cone beam computed tomography.
CR	Computed radiography.
CT	Computed tomography.
DAK	Detector air KERMA; this is the air KERMA at the entrance of the intensifier or the detector.
DAKR	Detector air KERMA rate.
DICOM	Digital Imaging and Communications in Medicine (a standard image format).
Dosimeter	An ionisation chamber coupled to an electrometer, a solid state dosimeter with lead backing, or a transparent solid state dosimeter (without lead backing) used to measure radiation dose rates.
DQE	Detective quantum efficiency.
DSA	Digital subtraction angiography—an imaging mode that subtracts an image (called a mask) in real time to remove over- and under-lying layers of anatomy. This is particularly useful to visualise the vasculature.
ESAKR	Entrance surface air KERMA rate.
FDA	Food and Drug Association (of the USA).
FFT	Fast Fourier transform.
Fluoro-store	The ability to store the last fluoroscopy run to a computer disk.
FOM	Figure of merit.
FOV	Field of view.
FP	Flat panel (x-ray detector type).
FPR	Fluoroscopy programmed radiology—modern systems require a period of fluoroscopy prior to acquisition before calculating the image acquisition parameters.

doi:10.1088/978-0-7503-3819-6ch7

FPS	Frames per second (note the terms pulse and frame are at times used synonymously in this document, reflecting that an x-ray pulse produces an image frame).
GSDF	Display grayscale calibration.
IEC	International Electrotechnical Commission
II	Image intensifier.
IITV	Image intensifier TV (system).
IPEM	Institute of Physics and Engineering in Medicine.
IRP	Interventional reference point.
KERMA	Kinetic energy released per unit mass.
LAO	Left anterior oblique.
LIH	Last image hold—the last image from a fluoroscopy run is displayed on the acquisition monitor.
LUT	Look-up table.
MDGN	Medical and Dental Guidance Notes.
MTF	Modulation transfer function.
NEMA	National Electrical Manufacturers Association.
NNPS	Normalised noise power spectrum.
NPS	Noise power spectrum.
PA	Posterior–anterior (bottom to top x-ray projection when patient is supine).
PACS	Picture Archiving and Communication System.
PMMA	Polymethyl methacrylate (a type of plastic/acrylic used to approximate human tissue for x-ray testing).
QA	Quality assurance.
QC	Quality control—the tests that are performed to ensure that equipment performs to a minimum acceptable standard.
RAO	Right anterior oblique.
RDSR	Radiation Dose Structured Report.
SID	Source to image detector (II or FP) distance.
SNR	Signal-to-noise ratio.
TO	Test object.
UQCM	User Quality Control Mode.

www.ingramcontent.com/pod-product-compliance
Ingram Content Group UK Ltd.
Pitfield, Milton Keynes, MK11 3LW, UK
UKHW051041120926
8556IPUK00030B/525

9 780750 338172